YOU AND I,
AS MOTHERS

YOU AND I,
AS MOTHERS

➤➤❮❮

A Raw and Honest Guide
to Motherhood

➤➤❮❮

BY LAURA PREPON

ABRAMS IMAGE, NEW YORK

Editor: Rebecca Kaplan
Designer: Diane Shaw
Production Manager: Anet Sirna-Bruder

Library of Congress Control Number: 2019939886

ISBN: 978–1–4197–4297–2
eISBN: 978–1–68335–828–2

Printed and bound in the United States
10 9 8 7 6 5 4 3 2 1

Abrams Image books are available at special discounts when purchased in quantity for premiums and promotions as well as fundraising or educational use. Special editions can also be created to specification. For details, contact specialsales@abramsbooks.com or the address below.

Abrams Image® is a registered trademark of Harry N. Abrams, Inc.

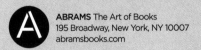

ABRAMS The Art of Books
195 Broadway, New York, NY 10007
abramsbooks.com

FOR BEN AND ELLA
AND
ALL THE MOTHERS

TABLE *of* CONTENTS

A New Kind of "Plus One"

I'M A MOM.

The same day I joined the motherhood clan, roughly 360,000 other women around the world also gave birth.[1]

Maybe you're a new mother. Or expecting to be one soon. It's also possible you're reading this book while your twelve-year-old does homework, your teenager practices on his drum set in the basement, or you've just gotten off a call to your kid at college. No matter ... I've written this book for us all.

Today is probably the best time *ever* to be a woman. We women can run anything: marathons, households, businesses, and countries. We can communicate at lightning speed, and our voices are finally being heard within our culture, shaping its future. Twenty-first-century ladies are not to be messed with . . .

And *still*, we are humbled by motherhood.

Which is weird, because we are neither the first moms on the planet, nor will we be the last. So how is it that something so ancient, commonplace, and downright universal remains so personal, powerful, and endlessly varied? Why is every woman so profoundly transformed by becoming a mother?

I know I was.

During my pregnancy, I was out to lunch with a girlfriend, and I asked her to share with me what she struggled with most as a mother. This was my first pregnancy, so I wanted to know from another working mom what to look out for. She peeked back over each shoulder, then leaned in surreptitiously, ready to share a secret. "It's . . . um . . . *hard,* girl," she whispered, as if she was supposed to have pulled off an A+ in Mommy class but had come up with a shameful C. I could feel her disappointment in herself. It was awful.

This scenario occurred on more than a few occasions: the whispering, the self-doubt, the apologetic tone. Not yet a mother, I could not for the life of me understand why. My rah-rah self thought, Come on! It can't be *that* tough. We've all dealt with plenty of stress before . . . you *got* this!

Little did I know, I was about to experience a shattering soul-explosion of my own. I'll tell you my truth, and not in a whisper: I felt *blindsided* by motherhood.

In the early days, I—someone who generally considers herself confident—felt insecure, clueless, and scared. I went from being the center of my universe to being displaced by a chubby-cheeked red-head staring up from my boob. I knew it was the natural order of things, but . . .

This was *big*.

One night, my daughter was asleep, and I sat in bed, crying. Ben, my husband, was listening to me patiently. "I don't feel like myself, babe," I confessed. I lifted my head and looked him straight in the eye to deliver what felt like the scariest line ever: "The woman you married is gone."

The words hung in the room for a couple of seconds.

"You are different now," said Ben. "You're a *mother*." He said it with such strength and nobility, it cut directly to my core.

I straightened my shoulders and lifted my head. I am a mother, I thought, and it's okay to be scared right now.

In that moment, I felt a shift: A version of myself was disappearing, and a new one was taking its place. And this new me needed new resources—stat.

Ever since then, I've been reaching out, asking questions, and doing research. I wanted to know what was

Why is every woman so profoundly transformed by becoming a mother?

happening to me . . . what happens to all of us when we go from woman to mother, and how to take care of ourselves in the best ways possible on this incredible, heart-squeezing ride.

And I've learned a ton: fascinating stuff about the female brain and how it changes during pregnancy and motherhood; the amazing role oxytocin plays in all our lives; effective ways of de-stressing;

how to maintain career/family balance; beauty and fitness tips; how to ask for help; and ways to keep the relationship with your partner strong and healthy once children are on the scene.

And because good nutrition is incredibly important (I wrote a cookbook called *The Stash Plan*, and I'm the daughter of a gourmet chef), I've put together some healthy, delicious recipes for you—some I've borrowed from other moms, and others I've created on my own, from quick protein fixes, like the perfect hard-boiled egg, to pho, a soup recipe that brings the whole family together—something that is becoming harder and harder to accomplish these days.

I continue to glean wisdom from experts and mothers who know the road ahead of me. I refer to them as my "Mom Squad," and they are some powerhouse ladies, including Mila Kunis, Jenji Kohan, Daphne Oz, and Amber Tamblyn, plus some other badass friends who work unorthodox jobs while bringing up their kids. I'll also share some amazing stuff from researchers studying the female brain and my own amazing ob-gyn, and I even sat down with a survival expert! They all offer fascinating facts and insights, and many of them share how they handle the daily struggles, uncertainty, and remarkability of being a mom. They give us tips on how we can take care of ourselves—physically, emotionally, and otherwise—as we do The Most Important Job on Earth. You will hear their voices pop up throughout the book, offering us their ideas and secrets and sharing their most humbling mom moments.

I'll also be asking *you* personal questions, offering you the opportunity to reflect on your own life and how it has changed since you've become a mom. We will also take a look at how other women mother around the world, getting a global perspective on maternity and considering all sorts of different ways of mothering.

We live in a culture where motherhood is most often discussed in the context of raising children and not the experience of the mother. For the first time, I was able to ask myself the hardest questions about my own unconventional upbringing, which brought me into confrontation with my darkest fears. The journey of writing this book has empowered me to confront the past, meet today's greatest challenges, and celebrate the deepest joys of my adult life. I hope *You and I, as Mothers* feels like an intimate, informative, and honest conversation between you, me, and my Mom Squad, as our real strength comes from dropping our defenses and sharing our truths.

Let's get started. I'll kick off this conversation with how it began for me . . .

CHAPTER 1

Ready, Set... Mother!

MY CRASH-LANDING INTO MOTHERHOOD

I was naked, wrapped in a shower curtain, on a cold, concrete floor. A long strip of duct tape bound my feet and hands behind my back, while a shorter one covered my mouth, rendering me mute.

I wiggled, trying to free myself, but it was useless. My captor, a man in black military fatigues, circled the small room menacingly. Frantic, I looked around at the five other women on the floor, bound and gagged just like me. He grabbed one of them by the hair, and she cried out in pain as he dragged her to the center of the room.

"Make all the noise you want," he growled. "No one is gonna hear you."

"*CUT!*"

Amob of crew members rushed into the scene. Duct tape was gently pulled from our mouths. I was lifted up, and my hands were freed. Through the melee of props being reset, duct tape adjusted, and wardrobe tweaked, I hopped to the man in black to offer him direction: "On the next take, remember the power you're wielding." He nodded, taking in the suggestion. "When you speak to us," I added, "It's scarier to say that last line like a simple fact: 'Make all the noise you want. No one is going to hear you.'"

I was directing episode ten of the fifth season of *Orange Is the New Black*. It was the last day of filming, and we had several scenes in a janitor's closet, where five of my fellow castmates and myself were being held hostage by the character of Piscatella, a power-drunk prison guard. Although I'd never had to direct myself while wrapped naked in a shower curtain with no use of my limbs, we finished the day successfully, and when I arrived home, I gratefully flopped into bed.

Ahhh.

The next morning, I could barely lift my head.

I was exhausted in a way I'd never been before. I was actually concerned about the depth of tiredness I was experiencing; my whole body felt like lead.

If being a director was this exhausting, I had a problem.

Directing was my lifelong dream. Even at seventeen, on my first big acting job—*That '70s Show*—I would study everything the director did, following him around, asking questions. Eventually, I tracked down a teacher at a film school near the studio where we filmed the show. He was the father of a friend, and when he saw how determined I was to learn, he arranged to teach me his directing curriculum in the evenings, after both of us had finished our day jobs.

When I finished the course, he ended up producing my next short film, and I was on my way.

But here I was, directing a prestigious project that more-experienced directors had vied for, and I was completely drained. Wiped out.

In an attempt to rally, I dragged myself downstairs to make what my husband lovingly refers to as my "moonshine." An epic, organic, cold-brew coffee made with homemade almond milk and simple syrup, this concoction never fails to get me going. I drink my moonshine every single morning; I even travel with my special coffee beans and my cold-brew machine. I love this stuff.

However, as I poured the coffee into my favorite cup, its aroma—which normally delights me—made me queasy. I did my best to ignore this signal and continued my usual cold-brew chemistry, mixing the ingredients *just so*. The ritual itself gave me pleasure, and I was hoping the brew would do its trick, but I could only take a few sips, and those I could barely swallow.

Something was definitely off.

I leaned on the kitchen counter and experienced the hot flush of fever. My muscles felt weak, my head was pounding, and I was woozy, but I was finally beginning to put two and two together: Someone on the set must have had a bug and given it to me.

I pulled on my sneakers and dragged myself out of the apartment to buy some cold medicine. Walking down my New York City street toward the closest pharmacy, I passed a vendor setting up his hot food cart, and the smell of sizzling meat produced a wave of nausea that made me lose my balance. I stumbled across the sidewalk and leaned on a building while I caught my breath. I did my best to act nonchalant for the passersby who were witnessing me doubled over and ready to vomit.

And that's when it hit me: *I'm pregnant.*

For a moment, the city seemed to come to a standstill, and I noticed only my own breath. *I'm pregnant?*

I reached for my phone, tapped in "signs of pregnancy," and saw that morning's itinerary read back to me: fatigue, nausea, headaches, flu-like symptoms.

That was me.

In shock, I staggered along to the pharmacy, but instead of grabbing Theraflu and Sudafed, I filled my basket with pregnancy tests. Wanting to avoid any possibility of misreading the results, I purchased every version: standard urine sticks, tests with digital readings, and tests with two-step digital readings. I grabbed a large bottle of water and started chugging; I was gonna need to pee.

As soon as I got home, I took all three tests and then laid them on the counter. I paced (as much as one can in the bathroom of a New York City apartment), waiting for the three minutes to tick by. I stared at the sticks intently for any hint of a sign. Then suddenly, they revealed their results like a Vegas slot machine: *pregnant, pregnant . . . PREGNANT!*

I sat in the bathroom, my vision blurred with tears. I cupped my mouth in excitement and awe. I had never even had so much as a pregnancy *scare*, and here I was, considering how my life was about to change forever. I always knew I'd be a mom someday, but I didn't think it would happen right that second. Ben and I had been hoping to get pregnant but not actively planning on it.

So this wasn't big news just for me . . .

I snuck into the bedroom with the digital test that clearly read *PREGNANT* in big letters. I turned on the bedside lamp and woke up my husband.

"Babe," I whispered, "I need to show you something."

I handed Ben the stick, and he read our fortune through sleepy eyes, which widened instantly. He pulled me into an embrace, over-joyed as the news rippled through him. "I knew it!" he said, with a huge smile on his face. "I *knew* it."

I bought every book about pregnancy I could get my hands on; I knew my body was about to undergo some big changes, and I like to be prepared. I read all the books, watched videos, and talked to friends. I downloaded an app that gave weekly updates on what was happening in my body, including comparing the size of my baby to a fruit or vegetable; that first week, she went from a pea to a blueberry.

I researched the best foods to eat while pregnant, bought books to read to my baby in the womb, and made a classical-music play-list to play for her through my belly. Having learned some power-ful nutritional wisdom in order to recover from health struggles in my twenties (which I detailed in my first book), I fired up a bone broth, pronto. I wanted to start nourishing my baby as soon as possible.

My pregnancy was pretty by-the-book—or should I say by-the-app?—as every week, my body mirrored the updates arriving on my phone: backaches, bloating, round ligament pain, heartburn, butter-fingers, crying . . . you name it, I went through it. All the books I'd purchased also covered these symptoms, so I felt assured that my pregnancy was par for the course.

Our birth experience also went as well as possible, given that the umbilical cord was wrapped around Ella in such a way that she was unable to descend fully. After eighteen hours of labor, we were faced with an emergency C-section.

Within minutes of that decision, I was lying on a table in a brightly lit operating room. My arms were out to the sides, tied to two planks, crucifix style. A blue surgical sheet was propped up at my waist so I couldn't see what was going on down below.

Ben was seated at my left shoulder, holding my hand as the anesthesiologist tested the numbness of my midsection. After a moment, the surgical team went to work, helping Ella make her way safely into the world. The precision, expertise, and care of my doctors were unparalleled.

I breathed deeply as Ben stroked my hair and whispered in my ear about one day visiting the coast of Northern California as a family. I closed my eyes as he described the gigantic redwoods we'd show our daughter. He sketched the sky, the waves, and the sun hitting the mountains with his words. As Ben was directing my mind, the doctor directed the surgery. "In a moment, you're going to feel a tug," she said. "It will feel like a little—and then a lot—of pressure."

I opened my eyes and looked at Ben. He smiled through his nerves.

"Okay," I said, not sure how much choice I actually had at that point.

My mind went silent. Just inches away, there were sounds, and pressure, but it all felt sort of distant. I held my breath. Seconds passed. The intensity in the room peaked and then released: Ella was out.

And then she *squawked*. That's the only way I can describe it. It wasn't a cry or a shriek. It didn't come with any particular feeling; it was simply a squawk of life.

Her first "hello."

The sound of her voice tore through my entire being. It woke up a part of me I hadn't known was there. I tried to inhale but was choked by emotion.

I ached to touch her, but my arms were restrained while my belly was being sutured, so the doctor handed Ella to Ben. I couldn't stop crying or catch my breath. He brought her closer to me so I could see her.

The mother in me was born.

For the next two days, we stayed at the hospital to be monitored after the surgery. After Ella's grand exit from it, my abdomen felt like a vacant room, where the original furniture—my organs—had to rediscover their places. I had to wear a special compression garment around my belly. Still, standing up made me feel like I was being ripped in half, and I doubled over just trying to walk five steps to the bathroom. I had to ask Ben to stop telling jokes, because laughing was downright painful. Even with all this, my doctor assured me that everything would settle and find its way back home, which it ultimately did.

The human body is a marvel.

The feeling of bonding with my husband, and this new life, is almost impossible to put into words. Together, we discovered Ella's perfect gripping fingers and impossibly tiny toes, and we gazed deeply into her eyes (when they were open). I felt exhausted, relieved, and madly, madly in love. It was pretty awesome.

And then we were released into the world.

Riding in the taxi home from the hospital, we now had a car seat between us, carrying our two-day-old daughter. Ben and I looked at each other, our faces weird mixes of fear and excitement as we started this new chapter of our lives. It felt like just a minute before, Ella had been in my belly, and now she was here, doing her little squawk, like she ran the joint.

It was surreal.

A few days later, I was sitting on the bed, staring into the middle distance, and being bound and gagged on a concrete floor was starting to sound good. I had been thrown into a type of sleep deprivation that blurred the lines of reality as I knew it. Sure, I'd pulled all-nighters before; I'd experienced brutal, twenty-three-hour workdays and long nights of debauchery . . . but nothing like this.

As those early days unfolded, I couldn't seem to figure out how to take care of Ella. My maternal instinct was there—I felt love beyond anything I'd ever known—but I was so afraid that I was going to mess up and she would somehow get hurt.

And on top of the fear was frustration. I am a prepper, a researcher. I like to study things, and I couldn't find a single book I could relate to.

No matter how hard I tried, I couldn't ace this. A horrible insecurity welled up and threatened to drown me; I felt crippled by inadequacy and self-doubt. I thought I had gotten rid of all that stuff years ago, and yet here it was, swallowing me whole.

Meanwhile, my hormones were all over the place; tears ran down my face, and they just wouldn't stop. My eyes were blurry from the constant stream of tears pouring out of them. I cried so much that I became dehydrated. I cried tears of fear that Ella might choke on her milk; tears from the pain of my C-section incision; tears of joy, watching Ben bond with Ella. I felt, for the first time in my life, totally out of control.

Other things started getting weird, too . . .

I used to pride myself on my memory: I could remember the names of waiters and waitresses from years before; entire scenes of dialogue were a breeze to memorize; I could recite the names of every single one of the two hundred *OITNB* crew members. Yet now, I was spending thirty minutes looking frantically for my keys . . .

The ones *in my hand.*

As the days passed, little by little I got stronger. I started to trust my instincts again. I finally realized that hormones are *real* and that they were responsible for so much of what I was experiencing; I wasn't crazy. Our confidence as parents started growing, and we figured out ways to get more precious sleep. Finally, when I was able to rest, cook, and move my body again, I felt my sanity start to come back. After six weeks of maternity leave, I returned to work.

Thankfully, I started to feel like myself again. An entirely different version of myself, with a completely different lifestyle, but myself nonetheless. I've finally realized there's no mastering this stuff, but what helps me most is sharing my experience with other mothers, hearing theirs, and continuing to learn as we go on this incredible adventure.

QUESTIONS TO CONSIDER

- How did you feel when you first saw your children?
- Which parts of mothering felt easy and natural from the start?
- Which parts have been more challenging?
- How have you seen yourself grow?

CHAPTER 2

How Were You Mothered?

LOOKING BACK IN ORDER
TO LOOK FORWARD

"Oh, my God, I'm turning into my mother."

You know the feeling. For me, it's usually when I hear myself using her phrases, like when I say that someone has "bats in the belfry" (an old-timey phrase meaning they're crazy) or muse that "hunger is the best seasoning" when a guest compliments my cooking. And when I crawl into bed with a glass of wine and a bowl of crunchy, salty treats (she called them "nibblies"), that's when I'm sure . . . *I'm turning into my mother.*

We are all affected by our parents, in many ways: from repeating their patter or habits, to the way a face is held; a quick response or lack thereof; the way you either chill a room or warm it up exactly the way your parents did when you watched them as a youngster.

My daughter, now a toddler, copies words I say, tries on my shoes, and wants to play with anything I have in my hand. She hangs out with me in the kitchen and raises her arms, saying, "Up, up!" until I pick her up and give her a better view of what I'm cooking.

She even watches my expressions and tries her own versions of them. I've been told I concentrate with a furrowed brow, a physical trait my father had, too. Recently, Ella looked straight at me and furrowed her brow, and I saw a glimmer of my dad. This perception of him—coming back to life through my kid—overwhelmed me with emotion.

Now that I'm a mother, I find myself thinking about how the parenting I received affected me, and still affects me, now more than ever. And it's not just the good stuff, but also the quirky stuff, as well as the bad. While I am a true proponent of "You are responsible for your actions" (a positive notion I gleaned from my mother), how we were parented, or *not parented*, affects us.

How could it not?

My mother, Marjorie, always looked like she just stepped off the set of *Dynasty*. She never left the house without her hair and makeup done perfectly, complete with false eyelashes and big hair with swooping bangs, à la Krystle Carrington. Her daily uniform consisted of high heels, black silk slacks, a loud patterned silk Pucci-style shirt, and a wide elastic belt with a large gold buckle accentuating her slim waist. Liberace-esque rings covered her hands, and as a child, I wondered how she could gesticulate with her slender fingers under the weight of them. I think that, because she grew up with nothing, she wanted people to know that she was a Doctor's Wife.

My mother had a Zagat guide that she would dog-ear and under-line. She liked to go to the top restaurants in New York City, try the dishes, then come home and perfect the recipes.

She would do her cooking into the wee hours of the morn-ing. Our household had no rules, and my four siblings and I often referred to it as *Wild Kingdom*. Although some of us needed more structure than others, I survived well with so much freedom, and I would often walk into the kitchen—after midnight—to revel in my mother's latest culinary obsession.

During her Peking duck phase, I found her standing at the counter, a large, plucked duck sitting on a pan in front of her. With elegant, swooping motions, she sewed up the duck's skin with a large needle threaded with cooking twine. "You have to sew up all the holes, so no air escapes," she instructed me as she turned back, concentrating on the task at hand. Her glasses hovered just above her nose, twine tied in a small bow at the bridge of her glasses, with the other end of the twine tied to a little hair clip that she clipped to the top of her head—a contraption she'd created so that her glasses never touched her nose, so no indentation could be left.

To this day, I wear lightweight glasses that don't leave marks.

Once she finished with the twine, she pulled a bicycle pump onto the table and stuck its tip into a tiny opening in the duck's skin. She told me to hold it in place as she pressed down on the pump. I climbed up onto a chair next to her and did as I was told. A loud *PFFST* sound filled the kitchen. I laughed as she continued to press down, the tip of the pump slipping out of the skin.

"Hold it tight!" she said, enjoying the moment thoroughly.

"It's slippery!" I giggled.

As she put the nozzle back into place, she instructed her midnight sous chef, "You have to get air *between* the skin and the meat . . ."

PFFST!

"That's how the skin gets crispy when you cook it."

She continued pumping the bicycle pump a few more times, then removed it to sew up the last remaining hole. She then proceeded to untwist a wire hanger as she asked why I wasn't in bed. "If you hoot with the owls at night, you can't soar with the eagles in the morning," she warned as she poked the hanger through one of the duck's eye holes and out through the other one. With a graceful nonchalance, she molded the hanger into a hook, off which the dead duck could hang. She pulled up the whole contraption, duck attached, checking it for strength.

It was quite a feat.

The next day, I saw the same duck hooked to my mother's closet door with a large fan blowing on it. She exited her oversized closet in her usual outfit, pulling on a long fox fur coat as I observed the duck gently swaying from the breeze of the fan. "You need to dry out the skin. That's how you get that signature crisp," she declared as she sashayed out the door.

My mother had passion. Her cooking allowed her to express her artistic sensibility, her creativity, and her joie de vivre. She was the most driven person I have ever known, and her stubbornness was almost inspiring. You want to see stubborn? Tell Marjorie she can't do something.

She continued making her Peking duck for five nights in a row until she perfected it, then moved on to her next phase: the Week of Caviar, every day of which she drove into Manhattan to Petrossian, a boutique renowned for its caviar, foie gras, and smoked fish, to get the finest beluga and sevruga. She would make blini—mini Russian pancakes—and then carefully pile the caviar on top of each one, finishing it off with a glamorous dollop of crème fraîche. I was nine at the time, so the whole concept of caviar was sort of lost on me, but I enjoyed the spectacle and my mother's intensity around it.

During Sushi Week we all piled into the car and drove more than an hour to a Japanese fish market in order to procure the freshest catch of the day. Marjorie would muscle her way in, standing shoulder-to-shoulder with professional sushi chefs, picking out her toro. She had confidence and strength and was never afraid to try something new. A quality I hope to pass on to my daughter.

Marjorie's mother, my grandmother, was all set to take her vows as a nun when she came back home to New York City for a visit. There she met my grandfather, who must have seemed pretty fantastic at the time, because she broke her engagement to Jesus for him.

Alas, he wasn't that amazing, because after fathering three kids with her, he bailed on the family during the Great Depression, and she was left with nothing but three little mouths to feed. With the pluck and courage she passed on to Marjorie, my grandmother got a factory job for Grumman making rivets for airplanes; she was a real-life Rosie the Riveter.

My siblings and I have many memories of going out to Huntington, Long Island, to stay with my grandmother. She would dumpster-dive for food and come back with iceberg lettuce and other odds and ends from her trek. We had become accustomed to a certain level of cuisine, so canned sardines and iceberg lettuce from the dumpster ("It's fine, you just peel off the outside leaves . . .") were a far cry from what we were used to. Looking back now, I can appreciate why my mother felt it was important for us to spend this time there. It also gave me a small taste of what she grew up with and empathy for how she was raised.

It's easy to look around at today's world and take our freedoms and conveniences for granted, so when I actually put my mother's life into a historical context, her spirit and boldness impress me even more. Marjorie went to Vassar, where she studied art history and drama before becoming an art history teacher. Given that she'd grown up with so little, getting into Vassar was a big deal.

An added bonus to college life, especially for a young woman who'd come from nothing? All the *food* available . . . and all of it *paid for*. There was more food than my mother had ever dreamed of. Who knew when there would be so much food again? She felt she had to eat it, and as much as she could. And of course, she ended up gaining quite a bit of weight.

It may feel like long ago, but in the 1940s and '50s, the role of the average woman was to become a mother and homemaker, while her husband was the provider. Just a decade later, in 1961, when my mother was in college, marriage was still a primary goal for most women, and how one looked was a very big deal: Twiggy was the face of fashion, the miniskirt and bikinis were popular, and it was a time of youth and rebellion. And because Marjorie had grown up with nothing, she craved the security of a successful partner.

But she also felt she needed to look a certain way in order to land a husband, so my mother ended up becoming a bulimic in college, desperate to lose weight. And, sure enough, when the weight dropped off, along came my father, a medical student. Naturally, the equations of "thin = finding a husband" and "thin = success" became hardwired in my mother and, thus, in my childhood household. The answer to all sorts of problems became "lose ten pounds."

When I was growing up, I was considered a tomboy, and I think I naturally rebelled against the pressure to be beautiful my mother put on my sisters and me. Although I could sense that something was going on with food in our family, I was too young to actually put together what it was. I remember watching a TV movie as a child called *The Best Little Girl in the World*, starring Jennifer Jason Leigh, about a young girl who suffered from anorexia and bulimia. With her life-threatening weight loss throwing the family into crisis, her father becomes hysterical and tries to force-feed her a peanut butter sandwich. She fights him off and bites his hand. That type of stuff doesn't happen in my house, I thought. That can't be what's going on.

I soon realized it was.

However, Marjorie expressed her dysfunction in more elegant ways. When I was struggling with my weight in my teens, she suggested, "You *can* have your cake and eat it, too . . ." I knew exactly what she was referring to, and I didn't like it.

"No, you can't," I snapped. I was angry that she felt she was above the laws of nature, that the rules of cause and effect didn't apply to her, and that she thought you could eat whatever you wanted and not gain weight.

But she also taught me, if you're going to do something, do it right.

"Don't use your finger," she said. "It's a dead giveaway; your face gets puffy, and your eyes get bloodshot and teary." I listened, both irritated and intrigued.

"You have to drink carbonated beverages while you eat, and don't eat heavy foods like Chinese or pizza. Those are too hard to get back up."

I learned that lesson the hard way, straining over a toilet bowl with tears running down my face, trying to regurgitate the entire pizza I'd just eaten: tears of self-loathing, tears from my obvious lack of willpower, tears from fear of weight gain because of the pizza brick in my stomach. Tears because I'd listened to my mother's advice.

After one of my bingeing sessions, I remember walking into the bathroom and seeing my distended belly. I thought how strange it would be one day when I was actually pregnant and looked like this because I was supposed to, not because I'd just gorged myself with food. Minutes later, I emerged from the bathroom with my normal belly again.

When I eventually did become pregnant, years later, I remember walking into the bathroom and looking in the mirror at my big, beautiful belly—filled with life. I felt Ella kicking inside of me. I thought about the abuse I'd put my body through, and my eyes welled up as I hoped the damage I'd done to my body wouldn't affect this perfect being growing inside of me. Praying she would be healthy, I suddenly felt ashamed, weak, and mad at myself. Mad at my mother for teaching me how to do it . . . and to do it well.

Thankfully, it's been years since I've binged and purged. However, to this day if I overeat, I can't help but think how easy it would be to get rid of it.

I was thirteen years old when my father died. We had been told that layers of fat were attacking his heart, making it difficult for the vital organ to pump blood. While he was on the operating table, the doctors, thinking they were removing layers of fat, were actually peeling away layers of his enlarged heart; they'd misdiagnosed him.

He died in surgery. Although he'd been sick, we certainly didn't think that we would lose him that day or that way. It was an incredible shock for all of us.

But I never saw my mother cry over it.

At the time, I considered this a sign of strength, and I wanted to be like her. I held in my tears as long as I could. I even went on a previously planned field trip to an amusement park the day after my father's death, because my mother felt it would be good for me. I rode roller coasters and walked through the park in a complete daze. But once I came home, I broke down, unable to hold it in any longer.

For years, I didn't cry at much of anything. Things that might make me cry—an intense movie, a relationship situation, a dramatic play—I would simply avoid. So once I became a mother, I was surprised that the human body could produce so many tears. It took me a while, and many talks with my husband, to realize that crying didn't equal weakness.

Marjorie instilled other concepts in me, like "If you want something done right, you have to do it yourself."

Propelled by this mantra, I went back to work as an actress soon after giving birth to Ella, and I found myself in the director's chair just weeks after that. I burned the candle at both ends, which wreaked havoc on my parasympathetic nervous system (more on this in chapter 5) as well as my milk supply. It took a panic attack and a brutal case of mastitis to make me realize that needing—and asking for—help didn't make me weak.

How I was mothered affected me in other ways, too, some of which baffled me until I figured them out. For instance, I found myself keeping my daughter on a very strict schedule. Any change in nap time or mealtime would cause a lot of stress for me, and I couldn't understand why. I finally realized that Marjorie's late-night cooking sessions had left their mark; having stayed up cooking until 4:00 A.M., she would often sleep during the day. Meanwhile, we kids would go to sleep in the evening, only to be woken up around midnight—for dinner. We'd lumber into the kitchen every night, greeted by multiple courses laid out in fancy casserole dishes like a five-star buffet. This was the norm for us at the time, and although I appreciated my mother's eccentricity, I later realized I wanted to keep Ella on a schedule so she felt the security of a structure. It dawned on me that, when I was a child, this lack of schedule—albeit free-wheeling—had made me uneasy.

I don't blame my mother for the way she raised us; for years I celebrated it. Her parenting style molded us into the people my siblings and I have become. As a woman in the 1970s and '80s, Marjorie was a product of the Second Wave of feminism, a movement that urged women out of their traditional roles as submissive homemakers and empowered them to explore their personal autonomy. Even back then, I knew my mother had had her own unconventional upbringing that also affected how she mothered.

Like every childhood, mine was a mixed bag. Although my mother was doing her best, given who she was and what she knew at the time, she had her flaws, and some of her mothering left me feeling conflicted and angry. I've had to work through that stuff. I've wrestled with resentment at times and am still figuring out how to pass on the good while leaving behind the not-so-good.

Sifting and sorting through my childhood, I realized that Marjorie didn't deliver lessons on right and wrong, but she did teach me how to cook the perfect hard-boiled egg without the yolk turning gray. I was never told to do my homework, but she showed me how to speak up for myself. I don't think she made it to a single PTA meeting, but she gave me permission to live with passion and to follow my dreams.

I also learned, from my mom, never to place the blame on others for my actions. I may be *influenced* by others, but, at the end of the day, I'm still responsible for the decisions I make. And I decide to take the good where I can get it. That means seeing that Marjorie did the best she could. And maybe I can do better.

So, how can we see our mothers' inexcusable behavior and also see their finer qualities? How do we separate the good from the rotten? How do we find nutrition in the things that may have wounded us? And—who knows?—what drives us to succeed could be the very care that *wasn't* provided. How you were mothered, and how you were *not* mothered, matters.

Five years ago Marjorie was diagnosed with Alzheimer's disease. The last time I tried to cook with her, she trembled just holding a spatula, not knowing what to do with it.

I do the holiday cooking now. Everything made from scratch, in roll-top chafing dishes just like she taught me, signature cocktails and all. Last time she saw me cooking for the family, she asked me how I'd learned to do all that stuff. I smiled at her and explained, "You taught me, Mommy."

There was a pause.

Then her face lit up. "Oh, my heavens!" she said. "I did a good job!"

I invite you to reflect on how you were mothered and how that might affect you today.

QUESTIONS TO CONSIDER

- Can you name three things your mother was good at doing?

- What are/were her best qualities?

- What strengths have you developed because of her, whether it was through her example or her failures?

- Which aspects of your mother would you like to transmit to your own kids?

- Which aspects of your mom are you *afraid* of transmitting to your kids?

- Consider your mother's story: her childhood, her struggles, her relationships. Does this exercise make you see her differently?

CHAPTER 3

You, Version 2.0, Mom Edition

EXPLORING YOUR
MATERNAL SUPERPOWERS

When I think about my life before Ella, it's as if I was a different person. Almost like I had a completely different existence on another planet. As new mothers, it's as if our lives are entirely reorganized, internally as well as externally.

I never expected this profound a transformation—and I certainly wasn't prepared for it—but soon after it had taken place, I knew I wanted to explore it. I wondered: How is it that simple hormones make me feel like I've entered another dimension? What activates them, and what, exactly, are they doing? Does this happen to everyone? Will there be other shifts like this?

Am I changed forever?

I sought answers from the experts, both medical and maternal. This chapter contains the insights of two doctors who spend their days studying the mystery of maternal behavior, and some members of my Mom Squad, who spend their lives living it.

It turns out that the brains of women who have children—whether it's through labor or adoption—are triggered by interacting with their baby's smell, touch, and cry to produce "mommy" hormones in such great supplies that they actually change the *structure of the brain*. And those neurological changes—many of which remain for life—produce a whole new set of priorities, behaviors, and maternal superpowers.

So, yeah, when I felt I'd become a new person after giving birth to Ella, I was right. Welcome to Laura, Version 2.0: Mom Edition.

Version 1.0 was pretty different.

For instance, I rode a motorcycle when I lived in LA. A Moto Guzzi V7 Stone, to be exact. It's a beautiful bike. I was always careful, never splitting lanes or zigzagging through traffic, but I loved riding at a breezy clip down the streets

The change felt bigger than any mere idea or decision.

of Los Angeles. There was something amazing about riding a bike, with the wind in my hair and the sun on my face.

I felt like a badass.

But once I'd given birth to Ella, I couldn't even *think* of getting on my bike. And even if I had decided it was a good idea, my body simply wouldn't permit it. Every single cell of my being said "no."

Nothing had stopped me before. My father, a surgeon, had referred to motorcycles as "donorcycles" because of the gore he'd seen them cause in the ER of the hospital, but even that hadn't quelled my appetite for speed. Obviously, it was *logical* that I didn't want to take physical risks after my life had become about protecting a baby, but what was the exact mechanism keeping my foot off the pedal? The change felt bigger than any mere idea or decision.

Well, according to the experts I've connected with, there's no question: I have been *rewired*. Did this explain what I called my "soul-explosion"? Had my brain been hijacked in a way I'd never experienced before?

As an actress, I lend my body and mind to other characters— sometimes for years at a time—so I like to think I have a certain degree of flexibility in the ole brain department, but it seems that no role I've ever played compares to Mommy.

I recently sat down with Dr. Pilyoung Kim, a researcher at the University of Denver and a leading scientist investigating the changes that take place in the maternal brain.[1] She gave me some fantastic insights.

"Rats really like cocaine," she said, which I thought was a pretty interesting way to approach the topic. According to neurological studies done on female rats that were *not* mothers, the reward networks in their brains really go nuts for cocaine. "But as soon as they have babies," says Dr. Kim, "rat moms prefer to have access to their babies over access to cocaine."

Wow.

She went on to describe what she called the "reward circuitry" in our brains, which responds to anything we find really pleasant, like food, drugs, and sex (and riding my donorcycle). Offered these stimuli, our reward circuitry lights up, and we get all excited and motivated. But women who become mothers experience a neurological renovation in our reward circuitry, making it respond most strongly, and above all else, to our baby.

"That's why we get up in the middle of the night and go to our crying baby," says Dr. Kim, "because we cannot *refuse* this. Our brain is telling us, 'Go and get some rewarding stimuli!'" It turns out that a simple smile on a baby's face, the smell of his head, the sound of her breathing—they all open up this neurological candy store.

And this reward system runs the show. As Dr. Kim says, "We can even feel kind of *obsessed* with our babies. Sometimes mothers say to me, 'It's something that I do all the time: I watch my baby, I think about my baby, I wonder if my baby is doing okay, whether I'm doing a good job . . .'"

I'm thinking: Check, check . . . *check, check, check!*

"And when you think about it," continues Dr. Kim, "it's really important in an evolutionary way that we have these patterns of behavior, because babies are helpless; they *need* our attention twenty-four hours a day. So we are designed to have this innate, strong desire to tend to a baby."

What, exactly, drives this change in the brain?

"Oxytocin plays a really key role," says Dr. Kim. "You've probably heard of oxytocin as the 'love hormone.' It is actually released by many different things; it can be gentle touch, intimacy, or if we see the baby smiling, or we hug the baby, it increases the oxytocin levels—not just in the body, but in the brain." And because the reward region of the brain has a high density of oxytocin receptors, this "love hormone" can increase the connections among the neurons in this area and really blow the lid off the candy store.

And the *last* thing Ella needs is me falling off my bike.

Another thing Dr. Kim said sort of surprised me, given how lovey-dovey oxytocin's reputation is. "High levels of oxytocin also bring about a really intense level of aggression," she adds, "so you hear, 'Don't cross Mama Bear!'" because women with brains bathed in oxytocin have a high degree of protectiveness for their babies.

OXYTOCIN 101

You may have heard a lot about oxytocin during your pregnancy or in childbirth preparation classes. It's also the hormone that surges during labor, causing the uterus to have contractions. Doctors, midwives, and doulas are all in the business of trying to dial up the body's oxytocin (or the synthetic version of it, Pitocin) in order to bring your baby into the world.

But your oxytocin production didn't start during labor, nor does it end there. Every time you've menstruated, your body has secreted oxytocin in order to make your uterus contract for the purpose of shedding its endometrium. With every orgasm you've ever experienced, oxytocin has pulsed to create uterine contractions as well.

But oxytocin has other dimensions. Beyond enabling contractions, oxytocin primes generosity, and in a study, researchers found that people given a dose of oxytocin were willing to donate 48 percent more to charity than those given a placebo.[2] No wonder mothers give and give and give.

Oxytocin also causes us to bond with others, and not just during sex. Whether it's with our partner, our baby, or a random stranger, if we are generating enough oxytocin in their presence, we will have warm, kind, and sort of *sticky* feelings about that person. We get attached. If you've ever believed that a one-night stand (who won't return your texts) was The One, you may have been in the throes of the oxytocin you generated during the encounter.[3]

And it was probably oxytocin that kept me off my motorcycle. According to Dr. Kim, "Our brain is bathed in this cocktail of hormones which activate the ability to protect the baby from any potential dangers. Oxytocin helps us to have this heightened sense of what baby needs."

I've heard this kind of thing from my Mom Squad friends, but the most dramatic description of the Mama Bear phenomenon came from a friend of mine who writes fantastic dramas. Jenji Kohan, creator of *Weeds* and *Orange Is the New Black*, is a mother of three and was refreshingly frank about how motherhood changed her: "I always thought of myself as a very peaceful person," she said, "but there was a realization [after having kids] that I could now *kill*."

I laughed. It was an extreme thing to say, but I totally got it. I would do the same thing to protect my child. And thanks to Dr. Kim, I now knew that the "love hormone" has an aggressive side.

"All of a sudden, not only do you become a mother, you become a potential killer," she said. "There's something amazing about that . . . I would take someone *out*. I would take *myself* out for my kid. It's this killer instinct that didn't exist before."

But oxytocin is not the only hormone in the mix for mothers. "There are pretty high levels of cortisol in mothers who've recently had babies," says Dr. Kim. "And cortisol is what we'd call a stress hormone."

That seemed like a weird combo, a love hormone *and* a stress hormone. But the answer to that mystery was staring me in my sleepy face: "For mothers to be alert—despite all the sleep deprivation—we think the cortisol helps. And we are trying to understand if it's also related to the high anxiety that mothers feel during this time," says Dr. Kim.

According to Dr. Louann Brizendine, a researcher, professor at UC San Francisco, and the author of *The Female Brain*,[4] there are even more goodies in the maternal superpower basket: "Mothers may have better spatial memory than females who haven't given birth, and they may be more flexible, adaptive and courageous."

How cool is that?

"These are all skills and talents they will need to keep track of and protect their babies."

Of course, this heady chemical mix explains a lot of feelings and behaviors that occur in moms during the first few months of motherhood, but what about over time? Once we have a 2.0 Version of our brain, do we keep it? Will we always be worried about our kids, watching their every move? Dr. Brizendine says that "the changes that happen in the mommy brain are the most profound and permanent of a woman's life. For as long as her child is living under her roof, her GPS system of brain circuits will be dedicated to tracking that beloved child."

SUPERMOM

According to *The Female Brain*, oxytocin also heightens a mother's sense of smell. We see it in sheep, says Dr. Brizendine. "When a baby lamb passes through its mother's birth canal, oxytocin pulses rewire the ewe's brain in minutes, making it exquisitely sensitive to its baby's smell."

Did you know that *you* developed smelling superpowers when you became a mother, too? Dr. Brizendine confirms that very soon after giving birth, human mothers, offered a selection of dirty onesies to sniff, can "pick out their own baby's smell above all others with about 90 percent accuracy." And that's not all. She adds, "This goes for her baby's cry and body movements, too. The touch of her baby's skin, the look of its little fingers and toes, its short cries and gasps—all are now tattooed on her brain."

When's Marvel going to make a movie about us?

So it eases up when they go to college?

Maybe not . . .

I met Dee when she was doing hair on the set of *Orange Is the New Black*. She had her first child at seventeen and supported her family by braiding hair in the Bronx. As she is now the mother of nine and grandmother of thirteen, I figured she'd know a thing or two about a mom's inner GPS.

"You have that bond with that baby—from carrying her—and you're connected," she says in her warm, husky voice. "I remember going to [Manhattan] on the bus from Long Island, and I had this sense of fear come over me, like, 'Something is wrong . . . something is wrong,' and I *knew* it was that [particular] child."

My stomach drops.

"I called, and, sure enough, she hadn't come home from school."

But thankfully, Dee wasn't sensing tragedy, just teenage rebellion: "She ran away and was hanging with a friend in the next town over!"

Phew.

"Even now I can always sense when something is wrong, and I'll call and say, 'You okay?' That sense never goes away."

These maternal intuitions can make us feel very connected to the Bigger Picture. Amber Tamblyn, a good friend, a great actress, and a founding member of Time's Up, describes her superpowers this way: "When your breasts feel your [baby] daughter in the next room and begin to leak; when your metaphysical being knows when your daughter is about to cry; when you have this borderline psychic capability . . . It's the closest I will ever come to understanding what God is. That power that is innately given to you: It's the instinct . . . the body's instinct, the mind's instinct . . . You can't take that away."

I had no idea that when I became a mom, I would be born into a whole new self, let alone such a badass one. It's time to appreciate all the amazing ways you've transformed into motherhood, super-powers and all.

QUESTIONS TO CONSIDER

- What were some other ways you transformed when you became a mother?

- How did this neurological rearrangement change your life or your relationships?

- Do you experience an inner GPS for your kids?

- How have your Mom superpowers evolved over time?

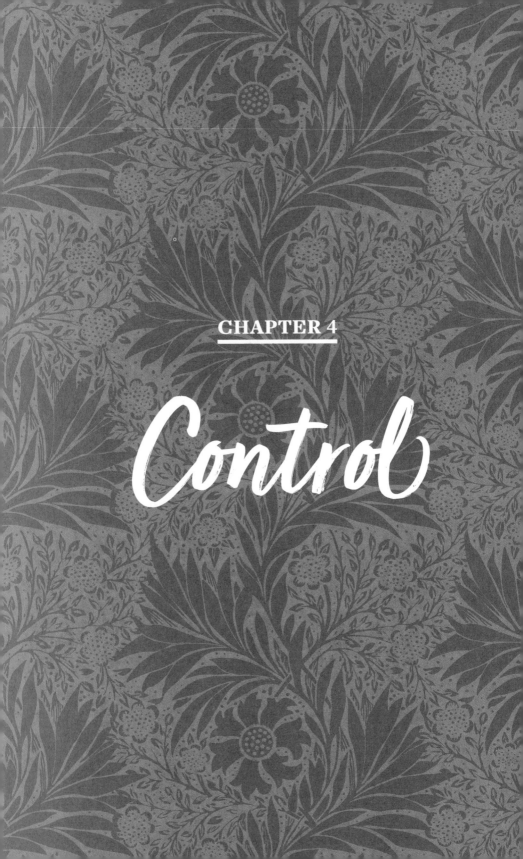

CHAPTER 4

Control

LEARNING WHEN AND
HOW TO LET GO

In the introduction I mentioned how, as modern women, we have more control over our lives than ever before. We have choices. We can continue our education or not, we can break up with a partner or stay, we can have a fulfilling career *and* be a great mother. Many of us enjoy a delicious autonomy within our lives, and as we make more of our own choices, the neural pathways of control (or at least the illusion of control) get deeply grooved into our brains and behavior.

But then motherhood comes along, and all hell breaks loose in the control department.

Near the end of my pregnancy with Ella, our ob-gyn, Dr. Lee Morrone, pulled Ben aside. "I'm worried about Laura," she said. "Women who are used to accomplishing a lot in their lives can have a tough time postpartum because so much of it is out of their control."

And, boy, was she right. If my inner Mama Bear had her way, she would control *everything*. I was used to having control, and motherhood demanded that I let go of a lot of it. And in certain moments, *all* of it. Friends assured me that I'd be able to guide my daughter's experience but never control it. I couldn't protect her entirely from pain, disappointment, or hard lessons, either. In fact, every mother I've spoken to, whether she was new to it or more experienced, has had to wrestle with her own loss of control.

When this happened to me, I judged myself . . . harshly. Of course I've experienced *regular* lack-of-control issues in life: problems at work, willpower around food, riding in a car or flying on an airplane. But this was a new level, and one I did not like. I felt like I was failing at motherhood, when I simply didn't know that this was an entirely new game, played by new rules, with new tactics required.

I had to learn to let go.

This chapter is designed to give you some practical tools so you can let go from deep inside. I have gathered wisdom from members of my Mom Squad on the topic of control, and every one of them, without exception, suggests we let go. Only by releasing the reins of control can we relax and tune in to our intuition. Only by unclenching our jaw, staying present, and breathing can we let the love flow. And as much as taking control might *seem* like the "responsible" approach to parenting, it can actually gum up the system pretty badly.

But letting go is not easy. Our instinct is to wrap our children in Bubble Wrap to protect them from bruises, heartache, breakups, not getting into the college they want, not getting a job they want, a love they want . . . the list goes on and on. But by recognizing what we do control and what we do not, we can reduce stress both inside ourselves and in our relation-

I simply didn't know that this was an entirely new game, played by new rules.

ships. From my own experience as well as that of my Mom Squad, being okay with giving up control is an active practice. It takes work to reap the benefits.

For me, tackling the issue of control begins with getting clear on what's mine to control and what is not. By taking this short inventory, I remind myself where my energy can flow easily, and where it can lead me to struggle.

Here is my personal control inventory.

WHAT I CAN CONTROL:

- My attitude (This includes having gratitude for work and family, being willing to practice letting go, and saying no to guilt.)

- The choices I make for myself (This covers just about everything I do—including my approach to parenting—and can be handled through prioritizing and preparation.)

- Nourishment for myself and my family

WHAT I CANNOT CONTROL (BUT CAN INFLUENCE):

- Other adults: my partner, other family members, my friends, and strangers. (This includes their behavior, thoughts, and opinions.)

- Change.

- My kid: her path in life, her thoughts and feelings, and what happens to her outside the house.

It can be daunting to remind myself of these truths, but when-ever I do, it helps me step into positive action, taking control of what I can. It's often helpful to take a look at some of those things we do have agency over. Let's begin with attitude, and a personal story that forced me to wrestle with mine.

When I started writing this book, I discovered I was pregnant again. Ben and I were ecstatic to be blessed with a sibling for Ella.

In addition to my regular gynecologist, we had a neonatal spe-cialist we would see for milestone scans: twelve-week anatomy screening, sixteen weeks, etc.

At twelve weeks, she told us that the baby had an elevated nuchal translucency or "nuchal" (a measurement of fluid from behind the baby's neck to the wall of the placenta). When this measurement is elevated, it can be a sign of congenital heart defects, spina bifida, Down syndrome, or other abnormalities.

Our baby's measurement was only slightly elevated. Like, 3.5 instead of 3, so our doctor wasn't particularly worried. We were already having genetic blood work done, and she suggested we add a test for something called Noonan syndrome, so we agreed.

Shortly after we entered the second trimester, Ben and I took Ella to the woods of Northern California to get out of the hustle and bustle of the city. It was the trip he'd described to me while he whispered in my ear during Ella's birth, and we were loving it. One morning, I received an e-mail from our genetics counselor: *Results are in! Call when it's convenient.*

I called immediately. All was clear. Negative for any genetic defects. Even for Noonan syndrome. What a relief. And it was another baby girl!

Ben and I embraced, and I cried as I thanked our counselor for the information. We couldn't wait to tell our loved ones about the new addition to our family.

But just minutes after I'd hung up, she e-mailed me again, asking me to call her back.

I felt a pit in my stomach.

Had she missed a diagnosis and was now about to tell me that something was wrong? I nervously dialed her. She asked me, very gently, to not share the news with our families and loved ones quite yet.

"Why can't we share the news?" I asked. "Is there something wrong?"

"No," she said. "I just want to get through the sixteen-week anatomy screening. Just to be safe."

I hung up the phone and immediately began counting the days until that screening. The wait was torture: eleven more sleeps until the screening, ten more sleeps, nine, eight, one more week until the screening . . .

The day finally arrived, and although we had an appointment to go back to see our neonatologist, my ob-gyn, Dr. Morrone, asked me to come in for some routine blood work on our way. We live about a half-hour drive from their offices, which are close together, so it made sense to do both at once.

We arrived at Dr. Morrone's office. We greeted the receptionist, who told us that Patty was ready to see us, which was a little weird. Patty was my gynecologist's sonographer. She'd scanned me many times during my pregnancy with Ella.

"Oh, I'm just here to have my blood drawn," I said.

"Patty is ready for you," she repeated.

Assuming Dr. Morrone had changed her mind and wanted me to get scanned after all, I said, "Okay, great!"

We walked back to Patty's screening room, and I hopped onto the table. Ben stood next to me, holding my hand. With Ella, we were always excited to have a scan; we loved seeing her progression and how much she'd grown.

Patty dimmed the lights and started scanning. I stared at the monitor. I could see the large umbilical cord floating around the baby.

Patty continued scanning, but her brow furrowed slightly, and I felt like something was off. I looked to Ben, and although he was smiling reassuringly, I could tell he felt something was off, too.

"Let me go get Lee," she said.

"What's wrong?" I asked.

Patty gently patted my arm. "Laura, I need to go get Lee," she said, and she left.

I turned to Ben. "What's happening?"

"I don't know, my love," he said, trying to soothe me as I sat up, panicked. "Let's wait for Dr. Morrone."

The next thirty seconds felt like a year. My doctor finally entered, greeted us, and instructed me kindly, "Lie down, sweetie, and let me take a look."

Patty returned to the machine and placed the probe back onto my belly. Dr. Morrone took one look and knew something was wrong.

"Okay . . ."

I burst into tears. I couldn't bear to hear what was about to come out of her mouth. Ben held me tightly.

"See that white line?" she asked, pointing at what I thought was the umbilical cord. "It's possible this is something called a cystic hygroma."

"What does that mean?" I asked, trying not to throw up.

"It means the baby's lymphatic fluid is outside of her body, in a sac."

From all of my research on the human body, I know lymphatic fluid is vital to the functioning of the immune system, so the fact that the baby's lymph fluid was outside of her was . . . *bad*.

Ben held me as I wept. Dr. Morrone went to her office to call the neonatologist we were seeing later that afternoon.

After a few moments, she returned. "I talked to her. We're going to have you get a fetal echocardiogram to make sure there is nothing wrong with the heart."

I couldn't stop crying. She gave me a sweet, un-doctorly hug.

"Laura, if the heart is not functioning, we may have to talk about some difficult decisions."

My body convulsed as I cried. She held me until I calmed down, then said, "Let's just get some information."

Within minutes we were in a taxi on the way to the hospital for the echocardiogram. After a painfully long sixty minutes in the cardiology department, they'd taken all the required measurements of the baby's heart.

"Everything looks normal," said the cardiologist, whom we'd only met an hour before. "You should go to your neonatologist and get your scan now."

Off we went to the neonatologist. We were feeling more optimistic. *Her heart looks good. Her heart looks good!*

Within an hour, I was lying in a third dark room. Again, Ben was holding my hand. We stared up at a large monitor as another probe glided along my belly. We watched like hawks as our doctor took measurements of the baby.

Then the lights came on.

"Lee was correct," she said gently. "The baby does have a cystic hygroma."

She pointed to a thick white line floating outside of the baby. "The sac runs from the top of the head down to the back of the knee."

She lowered her hand and looked at us intently. "The brain isn't forming correctly. The bones aren't growing as they should."

She looked at us as if to say, *Do you want me to go on?*

There was a horrible moment of silence.

"Is there any chance she might be okay?" I asked, girding myself against her response.

"Laura, the brain isn't growing," she said, her eyes full of compassion. "I'm sorry."

Ben held me as I cried.

She told us that further tests could be done, but it was unlikely the baby would survive to full term, and my body was at risk as well. After Ben and I discussed it with our doctors, the solution was clear; we decided to terminate the pregnancy by means of a D and C.*

I went over everything in my head again and again. Did I eat the wrong foods? Was I too physical at work? I had been filming the seventh season of *Orange Is the New Black* when all of this happened. Maybe I was working too many hours? Or did I do a physical stunt that jolted something the wrong way? I was so confused and angry at myself and my body. It was brutal.

When I reached out to my friends about all the internal conflict I was experiencing, I discovered I was far from alone. In fact, I was shocked to hear how many women had gone through their own version of this experience. When the topic of miscarriage or terminated pregnancies arises among women, so much loss comes spilling out. I found it deeply comforting to share with others who had gone through their own similar, heartbreaking events. Their stories had often been shrouded in secrecy. Some women had never told anyone about their ordeals.

* An abbreviation for "dilation and curettage," a surgical procedure to remove tissue from the lining of the uterus.

But that made sense. I, like they, struggled with deep feelings of grief as well as anger at myself. I felt like the loss we experienced was my fault, that I had somehow done something to cause it. And this anger I felt wasn't going away; it was curdling into resentment toward myself for not being able to sustain this pregnancy, for not being able to bring a healthy sibling for Ella into the world. I was mad at my body for not recovering fast enough, for not losing the stubborn weight, or for being tired all the time. The negativity was crushing.

I knew I needed to change something.

I turned to my friend Dr. Nicole Apelian, a scientist, herbalist, and natural wellness coach who teaches survival skills. She is that friend who can make a roaring fire without a match. Nicole survived in the wilderness of British Columbia alone for *fifty-six days*, living among bears and cougars. Her idea of a selfie is a photo of herself forge-welding metal on her property in Washington State.

I first met Nicole in 2017 when we relocated to Oregon for a movie shoot for Ben. He was cast as an army vet with PTSD who raised his daughter in the woods. Nicole was hired to teach Ben the kinds of skills his character would have needed to survive in the wilderness.

If that wasn't impressive enough, Nicole had survived a more harrowing personal adventure several years before we met her. In 2000, she suddenly lost the vision in her left eye. Under tremendous amounts of stress at the time, she had also been falling down frequently, wrestling with fatigue, and feeling as if she was fighting the flu. Concerned, her doctors sent her for various tests, and after an MRI showed lesions in her brain, she was diagnosed with a clear case of multiple sclerosis.

She was thirty.

"As you probably know," she tells me, now in vibrant health, "when you're told you're sick, you often get sicker . . . and it's not hypochondria; it's the mind-body connection."

That's why I'm introducing you to Nicole at this point. Her own experience of how our minds can affect our bodies is personal and real. She *knows*.

"I got sick. I got really, really sick. It happened fast."

In the following three years, as the MS progressed, it got to the point where she was using a cane. She had to quit her job, was often bedbound, and if she was even able to get up at night, she had to use a wheelchair because she was so tired. At thirty-three, she felt like she was ninety.

"Finally, I was like, *f#*k this*."

Determined to become a mother (something her doctors said would be extremely difficult), Nicole went off her Western medications and turned to Ayurvedic herbs, while also changing her diet, doing yoga, and doggedly reducing the stress in her life.* "I altered my lifestyle pretty significantly, and I slowly, slowly started getting better," she says, as I marvel that my powerhouse friend once needed a wheelchair.

In case you're wondering, yes, she had that baby. And then another one, both now healthy teenage boys. They make fires from scratch, too.

It was from Nicole that I learned about the mind-body connection and the power of offering gratitude.

---

* Although this worked for Nicole, always check with your medical provider before making important decisions about your health regimen. If you're interested in the details of Nicole's journey, you can check her out at https://www.nicoleapelian.com/.

GIVING EXTERNAL THANKS

"There is something hugely impactful about giving external thanks," Nicole explained. "The verbal 'thank you' for something creates an internal shift."

Although I had never practiced saying daily gratitudes, I decided to follow Nicole's suggestion. I started doing positive self-talk—out loud—to myself. I talked directly to my body about the pregnancy we had just lost. "It's okay," I said. And then I heaved a big sigh. "Thank you," I said, "for growing beautiful, healthy Ella." As I thought of her, my heart expanded for the first time in days, and I started welling up with gratitude. "I trust we will do it again."

"I forgive you," I said, letting go just a little bit more. "It's nobody's fault."

"I trust you," I said, as I remembered that about a fifth of all pregnancies don't make it all the way. "You have a natural wisdom," I said, and my body does; I could feel it in my bones.

Nicole had suggested that I connect with every part of my body, part by part, so I did.

Putting my hands on my head, I said, "I love you."

Moving my hands to my face, I repeated, "I love you."

At my chest: "I love you."

I covered my arms, my belly, my butt, my legs, down my whole body, and ended at the tips of my toes: "I love you." By the end of the exercise, I felt better. I felt connected to my body. I felt love for my body.

I started doing this exercise every day, and my physical and mental well-being improved greatly. Then I started doing "the talk" in the shower, and it became an ingrained habit. Not only did it help me cope with the loss of the pregnancy, it also helps with the daily stresses of life.

You can apply this exercise to anything, whether it's recovering from an injury or connecting with yourself after a lifetime of body/mind conflict. It's about being in communication with yourself, taking charge of your attitude, and appreciating what you have.

SHIFTING YOUR ATTITUDE

Our attitude is our outlook on things, and that's a big deal. Even though bad or scary things sometimes happen, and it's natural to feel bad for a while, there comes a point when we can choose our attitude toward the event (or person or place), and I find that positivity is always the better choice. It boosts immunity, releases endorphins (our brain's happy chemicals), and models resilience to my kid. Plus, it just feels better! But choosing positivity often involves a conscious shift in focus. It's on me to make that choice, and when I do, my whole family is better for it.

Sometimes I shift my attitude by aligning with someone else's. If I am stressed about something, my husband will remind me that we can choose our attitudes. He will turn to me with a smile and say, "How lucky can one family be?" He reminds me to be present and to not take things so seriously, that we are happy and healthy, and that we can be here *now*, in the moment. By seeing from his perspective, I can let go of that tumble Ella just took or the fall she might take tomorrow.

MAKING A GRATITUDE LIST

Since learning about expressing thanks out loud from Nicole, I've also practiced writing a gratitude list. You can do this daily or even weekly. I write down, using pen and paper, twenty things that I'm grateful for. I repeat many of the same things each time, but every time I write down those people or things for which I'm genuinely grateful (Ben, Ella, my health, our future children, our future grand-children, my career, our home, my friends, hot baths, nourishing food), my heart feels like it warms and my whole energy expands. It's such an incredibly simple exercise, with amazing and immediate results.

The trick is to be honest about what I'm *truly* grateful for and not to force things. It's okay if all I can muster is "this bed, this glass of wine, the *Planet Earth* series," as long as I'm telling my truth. When I connect with that inner truth, a powerful force begins to flow, and I start to feel better.

Equally amazing is the fact that writing my gratitude list seems to make choosing positivity easier and more frequent. I'm reinforcing positive neural pathways in my brain, and they're becoming my default mode. Give it a try!

PRACTICING LETTING GO

Letting go is about practicing an attitude of *allowing*. Sometimes I have to get out of the way and *allow* stuff to happen, *allow* my kid to be herself, *allow* myself to make mistakes and learn from them. Letting go doesn't mean we stop loving or showing up or nurturing, but it does help us stop judging, stressing, and sweating the small stuff. It's also practical, since every phase of life is temporary, and it helps us ride the waves.

Paradoxically, letting go is an active practice, and I ask my friends how they do it.

As the mother of nine children, Dee releases her stress to the divine. "I talk to God all the time. I ask for guidance, because I'm not perfect. When [life feels] out of my control, I just ask for guidance. Sometimes out loud, and sometimes I'll be humble and lie on the floor."

She laughs, at peace with her surrender.

"I'll be like, 'Look, I'm done. You need to take over.' I've had to do it hundreds of times, because it's not easy."

I asked Jenji Kohan, a mother of three and a show runner who has hundreds of people working under her, what her relationship to control at home is.

"At a certain point you have to give over. They [the kids] come in fully loaded. You can f#*k them up within a range, but they are who they are. I still try to control everything, but you have to have a sense of humor about it. I'm happy to give up the control for the joy. It's actually kind of a relief sometimes not to control everything. There's something really fun about saying, 'All right, we're doing *this* now!'"

When she can't be in control, Jenji knows how to at least shift the focus.

"This is something that helps me—as a storyteller—because kids (like most people) are narrative junkies. When they were very little, they [would] be freaking out about something, and I would say, 'Did you hear about the weird puppy?'"

Her eyes get really wide. "And all of a sudden they were like, 'What? A weird *puppy*?'"

She laughs, remembering her own kids' delight and curiosity. "And I would tell them a story. It's a great way to shift attention."

Daphne Oz is a chef, cookbook author, mom of four, and a wise member of my Mom Squad. "The worst thing I'm dealing with now—because my oldest is almost five—is playground anxiety. One day they're best friends with so-and-so, the next day that person doesn't want to play with them, or they're mean to them, or they call them a name . . . And watching your kids go through any kind of pain or problem is absolute agony. You want to protect them from everything. You want to go on the playground and lay some kids out."

I laugh, harder than I have in a while.

"But at the same time, like an immune response, you need to give your [kid] ways to learn on small battles so that she knows how to fight the wars. I have to let my kids out into the world; I can't be in control of everything. They need to figure out, in as safe an environment as possible, how to deal with things for themselves, so that when the big problems come—and I really *can't* solve them—I don't want them to feel helpless."

Logical, true, and still it makes me want to barf.

"The only way you get real self-confidence is by feeling like you are self-sufficient and that you can rely on yourself to get through good times and bad."

Jenji added something similar. "Intellectually, you know you have to let them fail. You have to let them make mistakes. You have to let them take risks. They cannot grow, they cannot flourish, they can't function unless they are given freedom . . . and with freedom comes *risk*. There is a temptation to be there all the time, and that's not good."

When I ask Nicole her take, she weighs in on the topic of letting go. "[Kids are] supposed to do dumb-ass stuff with their friends, away from their parents. That's how kids get social skills, right? They fight, they create a social structure, they play games—they do all that stuff out of view of parents. And that's the key. They're not *supposed* to be having adults watch them, because adults will intervene. That's our natural tendency."

Truth.

"But when we were young, we ran around in packs with other children, and we figured *our* stuff out. And we did some really dumb stuff, too; we probably hurt each other and hurt ourselves, but our parents weren't there to negotiate it. I feel like kids are around their parents so much now that they get stopped from doing that stuff.

They don't learn social skills, physical skills, any of that, if we're stopping their behavior."

Amber gave birth to her daughter about five months before I had Ella. Because she deals with many things before I do, we share a lot about our experiences. When I asked her how she handles this

---

COPING MECHANISMS

When we continually try to control the uncontrollable, we become frustrated. Conflict occurs inside of us, and it often leaks out all around us. When the tension gets high enough, we act in ways—or reach for things—to release all the pent-up energy. That's perfectly natural, but the choices we make matter.

A glass of wine after a hard day is one thing, but wine becoming Mommy's go-to may not be a sustainable option. None of us are perfect, and I bring no judgment to the table, but considering that parenting is a lifelong job, I want to touch on this subject, because it's worth taking a look at how we cope with challenges.

Here are some questions to reflect on:

- Are you getting frustrated because you're trying to control the uncontrollable? (Look back at the control inventory to find out.)

- What are your coping mechanisms?

- Have they become more frequent? When is your strongest urge to use them?

- If you were to surrender on an issue and admit you can't control it, would your coping mechanism be needed?

- How can you take care of yourself in a way that feels good and strengthens you over time?

loss of control, she plays it out on a bigger, global scale. "I realized I had to move the focus, to be less about keeping [my daughter] safe—because I can't control that—and more about modeling how to change the world that I'm afraid of."

We are sitting in my living room, and as Ella plays on the floor, I am terrified by the idea that I won't always be able to guarantee her safety, but I recognize this truth with a sigh.

Amber continues: "And I know that's a big, insane idea, but . . . I'd rather die trying to change the world. I'd rather sacrifice everything to try to change it than be complacent. I'm showing my kids that 'I fight! I f*%king fight for what I believe in. That's what I do. I hope you do that, too.' *That's* the message."

Beyond my attitude, I have control over my actions. Here are some ways the Mom Squad and I maximize this control.

MAKING CLEAR CHOICES

Having a child gives your priorities a vigorous reshuffling, and as time goes on, continuing to make conscious choices about how you spend your time and energy becomes really important. By making clear decisions and learning to say no, I can focus less energy on superficial things and bring more energy to me and my family.

It's not always easy. Many women (myself included) are die-hard nurturers, givers, and people-pleasers. Before becoming mothers, we may have been extending ourselves—quite happily—in multiple directions, toward many people and pursuits. Having to turn off some of those taps can feel hard or even induce guilt.

Believe me, I get it. I experienced crippling guilt when I returned to work after giving birth; every cell in my body ached to be home with my daughter. Focusing on work felt like a constant struggle against the new Mommy wiring we just talked about in the previous chapter. My brain, Version 2.0, kept craving contact with Ella, while the rest of me was directing an episode of *Orange*. As a friend of mine said about this work/career balance: "The juggle is real!"

Eventually, I realized I had to simply stick with my decision to work. I had to let go and be fully present for my job. I was far from perfect at it, but I did my best not to waver when the guilt crept in. I committed to focusing on work, giving it 100 percent, and to actively letting go of the guilt.

And then I came home and did exactly the same thing with my family, which meant I was fully present and fully aware. At home I dedicated myself to my partner and my child.

I've realized this requires a simple mental boundary—work is work, and home is home—that brings obvious benefits. It's another way of demonstrating that quality is more important than quantity.

Ben and I have taken this to heart. We both work, but we do our best not to bring it home, so we can be fully present with our daughter. If one of us is on a deadline, we take turns with Ella while the other one works, but it's our intention to let work be work and home be home. And although there are definitely times when we have to remind each other, it's made a big difference.

Amber weighs in with "I always go back to the same mantra, which is 'quality over quantity.' And that can be applied to anything: food, what you cook, the time you spend with your children, the time you spend with your lover."

My friend Angela Robinson is a writer, producer, director, mother, and serves on the executive committee of the Time's Up movement, as well as being co-captain of the WOC (Women of Color) group within it.

Given that Time's Up is specifically about safety, dignity, and equality in the workplace—across all industries—I was curious what Angela thought about the topic of work/family balance. She explained that in the entertainment industry, "a lot of times you're given this binary choice: Have a career that moves you to another city for half the year or limits the hours in the day you can spend with your kid—issues that really impact a family—or you *don't* have a career, and you stay with your family."

I've seen a lot of that.

"And the narrative is gendered," Angela continues. "If women with kids make that decision [to work], they are perceived to be sh#*ty moms who are so obsessed with their career that they're not there for their kids . . . but if they choose *not* to pursue that career, the narrative is that they 'don't have what it takes' or 'didn't want it badly enough.' Men don't get either of those narratives; they get, 'Of course he's going to take the job, and his wife is going to stay home and take care of the kids, and that's what he *should* do, and his career is awesome . . . AND he's an awesome dad!'"

I understand her frustration.

Then she smiles.

"Now, women are starting to [say]: 'You know what? That's f*cked up! Why do I need to choose this; why don't *you* guys change?'"

Mila Kunis, mother of two, shared a great tip for working mothers. "Never look at work as a negative in front of your kids. When I go to work, I say (excitedly), 'Mommy's going to work!' I never say, 'Oh, baby, I'm so sorry, Mommy's gotta go to work. I know this sucks.' Ever. [That way], they can aspire to have the same outlook on life and find a career or a job that's fulfilling and beautiful. Don't look at it as a negative."

Mila's on to something here. Having a working mother while growing up has been shown to be a very positive thing for children later in their lives. According to a major study done at Harvard, looking at data from twenty-four countries, daughters of mothers who worked outside the home eventually earned more and held more managerial positions than those whose mothers didn't hold jobs, while their sons went on to have more liberal attitudes about working women and contributed more to parenting and house-hold responsibilities.[1]

Of course, the transitions between work and home can be tricky sometimes. I asked Jenji how she handles it. "It's very hard to leave a bad day at work and be a mother again," she said. "For a while, I felt my kids were getting the worst of me. I would come home exhausted . . ."

I get it.

"What I found helpful was to be radically honest, because if you fake it, they know it. Own your s#*t. When you make a mistake—say something you shouldn't have, react too quickly—own it. We are human. And it's modeling for them—when they screw up, I want them to be okay telling *me*."

Being a working mother may always bring up mixed feelings. When I get home from a long day at work and Ella runs into our caregiver's arms instead of mine, it hurts a little. Or when I try to hug her anyway and she squirms away . . . But I can't let those things upset me. I have to remember how fortunate I am to have a care-giver I trust while I get to develop my career. I have to remember what I learned from friends who've walked this road ahead of me: Be fully present, for both work and family; quality over quantity; be honest about how I'm feeling. Because I know that, after I spend some quality time with Ella—undistracted—we will both relax, and our connection will be renewed.

Finally, when considering her priorities, Mila asks herself a simple question: "Is this worth me not seeing my kids for? Do I want to go to dinner with that person, or would I rather stay at home with my kids and my husband? [Parenting] changes the way you look at things."

I can relate. There is nothing more delicious to me now than spending time at home with my family.

"Time got put in perspective," she says. "Before, in our twenties, I looked at time as irrelevant. But you have a kid, and you *see* time, because you see your kid grow. And all of a sudden you think, 'Oh, my God, where has the year gone?' And your kid's one, and then all of a sudden, three, and you're, like, whoa, whoa, WHOA!! Pump the brakes! So I do find myself wanting to enjoy life more," she says, exhaling, "and appreciate stillness, because I find that things move so quickly around me."

So the next time you wonder whether or not you want to do something, or you're feeling guilted into doing something, ask yourself: Is this really what *I* want? Is this worth the time away from my family? Will this fuel me or deplete me?

PREPARING IN ADVANCE

After writing *The Stash Plan*, I was asked a lot about food and health-related topics. Since Ella came into the world, I've received even more queries via social media, at events, or just from people coming up to me on the street. They all want to know how I maintain a healthy lifestyle now that I am a mom. And I realized that one of my tricks, one of the basic foundations of my life, is preparation.

I am a prepper.

I use preparation to balance many of the aspects of my life. As an actress, if I don't fully prepare my scenes ahead of time (knowing my character, my lines, where to move), I won't feel confident about my work, nor can I be present for the scene.

As a director, I pride myself on my preparation. Whenever filming is happening, something will inevitably go wrong. You lose access to a location, an actor calls in sick, a snowstorm changes your whole day and you have to shoot completely different scenes inside versus outside. Because I am prepared, I feel freer to roll with changes, I get less stressed about them, and I can remain present for the unfolding of the *new* plan.

Angela, whom I mentioned before, has directed films and executive-produced shows from *The L Word* to *True Blood*. I met her, her wife, Alex, and their (then) ten-year-old son while filming the second season of *Orange Is the New Black*. Since then, Angela has become a mentor to me, and she always has very practical and effective approaches to both work and motherhood.

When I asked her about the subject of preparation as it pertained to motherhood, she shared this: "It's like prepping a movie. All these people come together, and you have to do this *thing*. So [with a movie], you schedule your time, how you're going to get things done in that time, and you *have* to get it done. You have to do budgets, and hours, and, as a director, you have to figure out how to make your day."

(To "make the day" is a filmmaking term that refers to getting all the shots listed on that day's schedule done.)

"And as a mother, I think you have to figure out if you can make your day. 'We have to go to a birthday party . . . we have to go to school . . . we have to get the black pants because of the school thing!' And if I can't do it, who is going to do it?"

She laughs.

"They used to say 'run a household,' and I never paid much attention to that. Then I was, like, oh, that's a *thing*. [Running a household] takes a lot of work. It's like a little mini-company. It's like an ongoing, ever-evolving, mini-production."

Boy, is *that* true.

As a mom, preparation is my best friend in the kitchen, and I love to spend a couple of hours getting major foodstuffs cooked so that meals for the next few days are easier. And I've even begun to learn that, although I can't control how Ella is going to experience her school or kids at the park, I can at least arm her with solid nourishment, so that she feels good in her body and can make the right decisions for herself.

Which brings me to the relationship between control and preparation. I've learned that good preparation helps me *give up* control. When I'm prepared, I can relax, be in the moment, and have fun. I prep so I can be present and take pleasure in the experience.

Whether you're a prepper or not, I encourage you to explore it as a concept and as a tool. What are some of the things in your life that might benefit from a little preparation? For me, I like to batch cook to have food ready to go in the fridge; I prep my work bag in advance; I lay out my workout clothes (so I have one less excuse not to go to the gym!); I lay out my kid's clothes—that always makes getting out of the house easier in the morning. I also like making lists, because they help me stay organized.

Keep in mind that prepping can often be done while listening to a podcast, hanging out with a friend, or talking on the phone. I live in New York now, and most of my friends are back in LA, so I like to use my prep time to catch up with them. I'll even prop my phone up on the counter and FaceTime with them while I prep in the kitchen. And because multitasking can also be educational, many times I watch/listen to *MasterClass* during a prep session and learn how the pros cook, act, write, direct, play music . . . you name it! Consider what can make prep time more fun for you.

It's time to get your prep on!

Here's a summary of the tools we've discussed:

- Giving external thanks

- Shifting your attitude

- Making a gratitude list

- Practicing letting go

- Making clear choices

- Preparing in advance

Dr. Morrone has been seeing patients in New York City for close to thirty years, has attended more than three thousand births, and was named one of New York's Super Doctors by the *New York Times*. I love hearing the knowledge she's gleaned—from both motherhood and her medical practice—and her viewpoint on control and motherhood has helped me: "You have to be comfortable with the lessons that you've given to your child. Things really do ultimately work out the way they're supposed to, and you know what? You can't control it! You can educate [your kids], you can guide, but there's a path that's been decided for them. And I know that sounds really cosmic, but I really do believe that."

>>>>>>>>>>>>>>>>>>>>>>><<<<<<<<<<<<<<<<<<<<<<<<

QUESTIONS TO CONSIDER

- When do you find letting go most challenging?

- What are three things you can control?

- What are three things you try to control but cannot?

- How can you make a change to better the world around your family?

- What is your actual priority list? What changes might you need to make to move closer to your ideal?

- In which area of your life would you like to be more prepared?

>>>>>>>>>>>>>>>>>>>>>>><<<<<<<<<<<<<<<<<<<<<<<<

CHAPTER 5

Stress

A MOTHER'S
DAILY CHALLENGE

Let's face it: When you're a mother, stress is a *thing*.

When I was seven months pregnant with Ella, I ran into a friend of mine who had just had her first baby. I eagerly asked what the hardest thing was so far. "The stress," she said. "Your heart is suddenly walking around *outside* of your body.* It's stress and worry you could never imagine."

Stress? I thought, I can handle stress. If that's the hardest thing she's dealt with so far, I got this!

* I had never heard this saying before my friend used it, but it turns out to be a version of a lovely passage by a writer named Elizabeth Stone. The actual quote is "Making the decision to have a child is momentous. It is to decide forever to have your heart go walking around outside your body."

And I didn't think I was kidding myself. I'm the kind of person who goes on stressful adventures on a whim. For instance, a few years ago, a friend showed me a video of a man paragliding around the beautiful Neuschwanstein Castle in Germany, after which the Disney castle was modeled.

"Ooh," I said, "that looks cool."

Fast-forward three weeks and I am standing near the edge of a cliff with a huge kite being stretched out behind me. My paragliding teacher approaches. "Okay!" he says in a thick German accent, "we are going to run as fast and hard as possible to the edge!" He mimes running with his index and middle finger along his other palm, and then his digits keep running *off* of his palm, into the air. "Then, keep going, with no ground underneath you," he adds, looking me straight in the eye. "And . . . vee *fly*."

As I try to process what he's just explained, he straps himself in behind me. I stutter as I try to clarify: "Wait, we run into the air?"

"Run!" he yells, and before I know it, we are bolting toward the edge of the cliff, the kite just barely picking up wind behind us.

"*Faster!*" he shouts in my ear from behind.

I move as quickly as I can. I feel like I am running in water—against a wicked current—with the edge of the cliff approaching rapidly.

Suddenly, my feet run over the edge, into the air, and we sail off into the sky, making a graceful swoop, corkscrewing around the castle just like I'd seen in the video only a few weeks before.

It. Is. Awesome.

I loved my forays into the world of high-stress fun. I've hiked to the summit of Mount Kilimanjaro without training (which I wouldn't recommend!), jumped out of planes, swum with sharks, and in my twenties I loved high-stakes poker so much, I ended up being nicknamed the "Home-Game Honey" on the cover of a poker magazine and played at the World Series of Poker . . . twice.

So, yeah, I thought I was good with stress.

But after my daughter was born, I experienced a kind of stress and anxiety I'd only ever heard about. I would catch myself holding my breath for what felt like minutes on end, bracing myself for something bad to happen. My hair started falling out, my chest was tight, and when I did breathe consciously, my lungs felt like they couldn't fill completely.

Just the *thought* of taking Ella out of the house made my heart race. Everything was a threat: The sound of a fire engine blaring was a personal attack on my family; I feared that Ben carrying her against his chest would make her overheat; strangers suddenly looked suspicious. This new vigilance was so intense that I began misreading things: A light switch turning on in the next room seemed like a warning, something I hadn't planned for, something that

> *After my daughter was born, I experienced a kind of stress and anxiety I'd only ever heard about.*

was going to hurt my daughter. Of course the sleep deprivation only made things worse, and the littlest thing would cause me to conjure gale force winds and hurricanes and the feeling that I was being swallowed up by the sea, when in reality . . . Ella had the hiccups.

Early on, breastfeeding was stressful as well. I got the hang of it enough to get my daughter the nourishment she needed, but it definitely didn't come easily. One day while nursing, I started experiencing nerve pain. It felt like electric shocks shooting from my nipple straight up into my armpit. It was awful, but I brushed it off, hoping Ella had just gotten a weird latch.

The next day, I woke up and knew I needed to go to the doctor.

The cab ride uptown was the worst trip I've ever taken. Every bump and pothole felt like an assault on my boob. I made my hands into a makeshift sports bra, holding my chest as tightly as I could, as we weaved through the turbulent streets of New York. I'm sure the driver found it interesting!

I got to the doctor's office and couldn't stop crying as I waited for Dr. Morrone. The pain was excruciating. I couldn't catch my breath. My chest was tight. I started to panic, and my throat closed up.

When Dr. Morrone arrived and saw my anguish, she immediately had me lie down and tried to get me to relax. I writhed around, the paper on the table crinkling wildly beneath me. She could barely touch my boob, it was so swollen and red. The pain was on par with trying to walk to the bathroom after my cesarean section.

She knew right away it was mastitis. Needless to say, that didn't help my stress level. The pain and agitation had brought me to a full-blown panic attack, a first for me.

But the stress didn't end there.

A few days later, I was in that groggy state between waking and sleep when I heard a *crack!* I felt something small and hard in my mouth. In my stupor, I removed whatever it was and went back to sleep. The next day my husband told me I was grinding my teeth during the night.

"I don't grind my teeth," I scoffed, although my jaw was sore.

I lurched out of bed and plodded into the bathroom. As I started to brush my teeth, I noticed that half of my left incisor was missing! Apparently I *did* grind my teeth. Enough to crack a tooth in half!

Between the hypervigilance, panic attacks, and broken tooth, I knew I needed to get a handle on my stress.

WHAT IS STRESS?

Luckily, I did quite a bit of research on stress for my first book, so I was familiar with how it works. The stress response is a lifesaving biological function allowing us to run from predators or take down the threat. This is what we call the fight-or-flight response. In recent years, scientists have added "freeze" to the list, because some animals play dead when a predator is sniffing about.[1] So, if your initial response to a high-stress situation is to feel rendered immobile, you're not alone.

These responses were really handy back in the day.

Imagine you see a saber-toothed tiger. Your brain freaks out and tells the hypothalamus (a specific area of your brain) to send a signal to your adrenal glands (located above your kidneys) to release adrenaline and cortisol, putting you on high alert. These hormones, in turn, cause your liver to produce extra blood sugar, also known as glucose. Glucose is the principal source of energy for all of the cells in our body, so when cortisol sends a shot of glucose into your blood, you get the extreme boost of energy required to either fight the tiger or to hightail it outta there!

This shifting into survival mode means you are functioning from your sympathetic nervous system. Although "sympathetic" sounds like it should entail a softer, gentler response, don't be fooled. In this mode, your body will increase your heart rate, send blood rushing to major muscles groups, cause blood vessels to constrict to divert more oxygen to your muscles, and make your lungs pump more oxygen so you can get oxygen-rich blood to your muscles. It's an incredible and highly sensitive system.

However, this mechanism is meant to *turn off* after the stressful situation ends. When the tiger gets tired or finds easier prey, and you climb back down from the tree you scaled up, the hypothalamus should tell all systems to chill out and return to the status quo. Your body is designed to shift back to the *para*sympathetic nervous system, the one that reestablishes equilibrium in the body. Often described as the rest-and-digest response, it is the parasympathetic nervous system that allows us to sleep, heal our bodies, digest our food, have good sex, laugh, play with our kids, and make cave paintings—in other words, live our lives.

But this doesn't always happen.

Although there aren't any actual saber-toothed tigers around anymore, there are a million and one things in our world that cause

TEND-AND-BEFRIEND

It may sound simple, but caring for others—or receiving care from them—may be the most effective, and easiest, way to deal with stress.

We've already discussed the fight-flight-freeze response to stress, but it turns out that's not the entire picture. In 2000, researchers at UCLA discovered an additional—and intuitive—way of responding to stress that women often revert to quite naturally. They named it the tend-and-befriend response.[2]

"Tend" refers to taking care of our children (or other vulnerable parties). You may have noticed that by nurturing and protecting your kids, not only do you calm them, but you soothe yourself as

well. Oxytocin naturally lowers cortisol levels, so by connecting in a loving way to your children, you feel better.

"Befriend" means seeking out our social group for mutual support. When faced with difficulties, it seems that many women prefer to talk things out rather than isolate themselves. And again, among the many pleasures we get from connecting with a friend, our oxytocin gets flowing during a good phone call or a leisurely latte. So that impulse to call someone in the heat of a stressful situation or to download later to a friend? The need to hug your kid? They're ancient, therapeutic responses, and they work wonders.

stress, external and internal. Our workaholic culture values constant *doing*. Keeping up with the bills can cause unremitting pressure. We jack ourselves up on caffeine and other, stronger stimulants; we often live in stressful environments with scary bosses, rude strangers, screeching subway trains, and some very real threats to our physical safety. And let's not forget the news: Just watching five minutes of the headlines will send you directly into the fight-flight-freeze response. Long before kids come into the mix, there is enough in this world to keep you on high alert 24/7. And that isn't even taking into account *internal* stressors: fighting infections, yeast, bacteria, etc., which have their own impact on us.

So, yeah, there may not be a saber-toothed tiger in my living room, but my hypothalamus doesn't know that.

When stress becomes chronic, it causes real problems. Your heart will work too hard for too long. If your blood pressure rises, so does your risk of stroke or heart attack. During times of stress, the immune system becomes temporarily suppressed, which lowers your ability to fight off viruses like the common cold, flu, or a herpes outbreak, as well as nasty bacterial infections. Suppressed immunity can also worsen autoimmune conditions like rheumatoid arthritis, multiple sclerosis, lupus, and Hashimoto's disease. It even raises our risk of developing many cancers.

If you wrestle with insomnia, anxiety, or depression, your internal pressure and tension probably play a role in your suffering. So, as much as we might sometimes like to wear our stress as a Maternal Medal of Honor, it can do real damage over time.

Wait. There's more. Sorry if this stresses you out . . .

Chronic stress also causes the immune system to become increasingly desensitized to cortisol, and since inflammation is partly regulated by cortisol, this decreased sensitivity heightens the inflammatory response and allows inflammation to get out of control. I wrestled with chronic inflammation for years, and it underlies a host of conditions, including bloating, skin issues, joint stiffness, headaches, diabetes, and heart disease, and it is also implicated in many types of cancer. It's even associated with accelerated aging.

Stress is also far from ideal for our sex lives. It's not unusual for mothers to lose their desire to have sex when under constant stress. Chronic stress in men can also lead to erectile dysfunction and a general loss of libido. So if you want to address the situation between the sheets, stress needs to be addressed . . . so you can de-stress, undress . . .

And have some sex!

If all that doesn't convince you to learn how to rev down your inner engine, consider this: Stress can also make you fat.

When we are stressed out and the sympathetic nervous system is revved up, cortisol not only increases your appetite, but also causes your body to store fat. And why would you store fat? Well, when cortisol sends more glucose into the bloodstream, insulin is the hormone that ushers it into the cells of your muscles to be used as energy. But insulin is *also* the hormone that stores glucose as fat. So when there is extra glucose left unused by the muscles, it gets packed away on your thighs or hips, so you have extra reserves in case you need it for later. And unfortunately, our bodies can't distinguish between physical threats and urgent e-mails, so a full in-box means there's a whole lot of glucose being released, with nowhere to go but your fat cells.

The takeaway: Learning how to relax is not just good for your health, your relationships, and your peace of mind; it can also help you fit into your favorite clothes again.

How do we bring ourselves back to the parasympathetic nervous system (rest-and-digest) more often and more easily? How do we help ourselves really enjoy our kids, our partners, and our lives?

When I realized I had to get a handle on my stress, I reached back out to my Mom Squad.

You met Nicole in the previous chapter. After bringing herself back to vibrant health following a multiple sclerosis diagnosis and being wheelchair-bound at the age of thirty, she was able to get off all of her meds, set her MS into dormancy, and have a thriving life with two healthy sons.

When I met Nicole, I was seven months pregnant with Ella. I was able to be in some of her wilderness training sessions with Ben and take in some of the knowledge she was imparting. She taught him how to build a waterproof shelter out of his surroundings in the woods, how to "range out" from his shelter to gather resources—all the things required to meet his basic needs. She even taught him how to make a fire from scratch and how to search for edible and medicinal plants.

Of all the things I learned from Nicole—the mind-body connection, external thanks—one of the first was an easy and enjoyable tool for reducing stress.

CONNECTING WITH NATURE

We all know that hanging out in nature is pleasurable, but it's also been scientifically proven to calm us down. When researchers from the University of East Anglia assessed the data from over 140 studies—involving a total of 290 million people in over 20 countries—their conclusion was definitive: "People living closer to nature . . . had reduced diastolic* blood pressure, heart rate, and stress. In fact, one of the really interesting things we found is that

---

* The diastolic is the second, lower number of your two-number blood-pressure reading. It's the pressure in your arteries as your heart rests between beats.

exposure to green space significantly reduces people's levels of salivary cortisol—a physiological marker of stress."[3]

They also proved that being in nature is downright healing. "We found that spending time in, or living close to, natural green spaces is associated with diverse and significant health benefits. It reduces the risk of type 2 diabetes, cardiovascular disease, premature death, and preterm birth, and increases sleep duration."

The late Oliver Sacks, writer and neurologist, put it in a lovely way: "As a writer, I find gardens essential to the creative process; as a physician, I take my patients to gardens whenever possible. All of us have had the experience of wandering through a lush garden or a timeless desert, walking by a river or an ocean, or climbing a mountain and finding ourselves simultaneously calmed and reinvigorated, engaged in mind, refreshed in body and spirit."

In order to experience this kind of connection, Nicole recommends finding a "sit spot." This is something anyone, anywhere, can do, whether you live in an urban or rural area.

FIND YOUR SPOT

This can be on a park bench, in the depths of the woods, or even on the porch of your own home. Just make it outside. It's best if there are some natural things to look at or listen to; a tree, a bird feeder, and some neighborhood cats are a fine start.

SIT THERE DAILY

Even if it's just for five minutes, by going to your sit spot daily, you'll be training your nervous system to slow down. Remember to turn your phone off completely (or leave it at home).

RELAX AND SIMPLY NOTICE THINGS

This is what Nicole refers to as a "soft skill," something that helps us reconnect with nature in an easy and enjoyable way. By spacing out in your sit spot, she says: "You see changes, seasonal changes; you see the robin building its nest; you hear the crows making a noise and think, 'Oh, what are they talking about?'"

As she describes it, I can almost hear them.

"Maybe you see a cat pass by," she says, "and you just put another *connection* together." And this connection is primal, the stuff of our DNA. "Now you have a relationship with that particular bird making a nest—not with robins in general but with *that* robin. That string [of connection] forms a rope, and those ropes of connection are important. They're what give you an overwhelming feeling of connecting with nature."

My family lives near a small park, and I will often sit down on a bench there with my daughter and just look at the trees, noticing how they've changed in the previous weeks. Then I'll catch a glimpse of a squirrel darting and twitching and gathering things for his survival. And the clouds moving above us become part of our nature movie. I also take real delight in seeing what Ella notices as she discovers new things about the world. Sitting in our nature spot brings a simple yet profound joy.

LEARNING TO BREATHE

This may sound odd. We've been breathing our whole lives. But the way we breathe affects so many things. And although breathing is involuntary most of the time, we *can* also direct it consciously, altering all sorts of functions in the body, including stress levels.

When I was working on *That '70s Show* as a teen and young adult, the director would tell me again and again that I needed to learn how to breathe to support my voice. I knew he was right, because if I had to do a scene with a raised voice, I couldn't talk for days afterward. But I was young, and I never really understood the importance of it.

Still, I started to pay a little more attention, but, honestly, it wasn't until I became a mother and found myself holding my breath for what felt like minutes at a time that I gave breath its due respect. And a panic attack made me really understand my relationship to air, because my throat closed up, and I couldn't get any into my lungs!

These days I'm starting to recognize that how I breathe affects my mind, my mood, and my health. From the deep breaths of yoga to the box breathing technique coming up, I've learned that how air flows into my body has the power to rev me up or calm me down. And I talk a lot about breath with my family now. Even with Ella, two of the first words she learned were "inhale" and "exhale" as I showed her how to take big breaths into her body.

There are many ways of focusing on your breath to calm yourself down. Below are a few techniques I've learned from specialists as well as members of my Mom Squad that you can easily fit into your day.

BOX BREATHING

While my husband was filming a movie called *Lone Survivor*, he played a Navy SEAL named Matthew Axelson. It was based on the true story of SEAL Team 10 deployed on a surveillance mission in Afghanistan that went horribly wrong.

While Ben was preparing for this role, he was able to train with—and learn from—real SEALs. They shared a technique they use to stay calm when under attack or when they need to focus on an objective. It's called box breathing, based on the idea that a box (a two-dimensional box) has four sides. The technique is simple but instantly focuses the mind and calms the body.

- Inhale to a count of four.

- Hold for a count of four.

- Exhale to a count of four.

- Hold for a count of four.

- Repeat.

This technique is great for a day that has a lot going on; I do it in the car on the way to my next meeting, or at work, or even hanging out at home if I need to settle myself.

Box breathing is just one form of what's called diaphragmatic breathing (controlled deep breathing), and research shows it really works. When observing participants in a 2017 study, researchers found that those who did diaphragmatic breathing had significantly lower cortisol levels after practicing their techniques than those in a control group who breathed normally. A 2009 study also showed that five minutes of deep breathing, repeated over thirty days, helped lower anxiety in pregnant women experiencing signs of preterm labor.

Here are two more breathing techniques you can try.

ALTERNATE-NOSTRIL BREATHING

Practiced for centuries by yogis but recently brought into the lime-light by Hillary Clinton as one of the ways she de-stressed after her election loss, alternate-nostril breathing has been shown to lower heart rate and blood pressure and to increase oxygen flow.[4] It goes like this:

- Get into a comfortable upright position and close your eyes.

- Press your right thumb against your right nostril.

- Inhale deeply through left nostril.

- Press your ring finger against your left nostril, so that both nostrils are closed.

- Hold your breath for a moment.

- Release your thumb and exhale completely through the right nostril.

- Repeat but in reverse, inhaling through the right nostril while holding the left, closing both nostrils for a moment, and then exhaling through the left nostril.

- Repeat for a few minutes.

Because alternate-nostril breathing requires a bit more focus, and since it involves constant touching of my nose, I prefer to do it in private.

YOGA BREATHING

If you practice yoga, the breathing you do in class will also provide major stress reduction. In a recent study, participants were asked to do deep yogic breathing exercises while another group sat quietly and read. The heavy breathers saw a decrease in three stress-related biomarkers, while the readers experienced none.[5] I love to read for relaxation, but I might need to add some de-stressing breaths to rev down even more.

Yoga is a great overall stress reducer, and I highly recommend it. Even ten minutes a day of yoga poses centers my mind, strengthens my body, and calms me down. And it also has a bonus quality: A study done at the University of Utah showed that yoga is so good at helping us regulate the stress response, it reduces sensitivity to pain![6]

CONNECTING WITH A FRIEND

We all know intuitively that confiding in a safe and empathetic friend makes us feel better, but now the science backs it up as the tend-and-befriend response. Just the sound of a loved one's voice can lower our stress hormones and get our oxytocin flowing. Confiding in someone we trust also provides a great opportunity to get some perspective and maybe even some good advice. I love to call my friends back in LA for long talks or get together with my sisters for dinner. There's nothing like a latte with a girlfriend, even if we do have the kids running around. It nourishes us both. More on this in chapter 9.

GROUNDING YOURSELF

I recently spoke with Jill Blakeway, an acupuncturist, energy healer, mother, and owner/founder of the Yinova Center in New York City. She's written two books that I am a fan of, *Energy Medicine* and *Sex Again*, and has treated both male and female patients for over twenty years.

As a working mother, I am often pulled in many different directions, which can leave me feeling stressed and depleted. I asked Jill, as an energy worker who juggles a thriving practice, a busy family, and being an author, how she protects her energy.

"I learned to ground and center myself," she says. "In energy work, they often tell you, 'You have to protect yourself.' That's very fear-based. But the truth is, you don't have to protect yourself; you need to stay grounded and then pull energy into yourself."

I ask her to show me.

"When I ground myself, I literally put my feet on the ground."

I jump up to do it with her. I need some grounding, and I want to make sure to get it right. I stand across from Jill. She smiles and continues.

"I bend my knees. I tip my pelvis forward . . ."

I follow suit.

"Feet shoulder-width apart. Knees slightly bent, pelvis forward, you feel yourself ground."

And I do. My whole posture and sense of balance has shifted with just these tiny adjustments. I feel connected to my feet, the floor, the earth.

"Then imagine a big anchor chain going down into the center of the earth, and take a breath and push that chain right down into the center of the earth; you feel yourself getting heavier, and you wrap it around the molten core at the center of the earth in your mind. Then put your shoulders back and your head up."

I feel taller and yet more grounded. More powerful.

Jill can see the shift in me. "Stay in this stance, and imagine white light—energy—pouring into your body from your crown chakra (top of head), and flood your body with that light. That's your own spiritual light. That's you connecting to Source."

It feels fantastic.

Since learning it, I've used this technique several times at work when things feel chaotic or are not going according to plan. By centering and grounding myself, I'm able to stay present under quickly shifting circumstances.

Try it yourself!

MEDITATION

The majority of mothers I interviewed for this book meditate in one way or another. And when I say "meditate," I mean they practice some version of calming and focusing their minds—no matter their religious or spiritual beliefs.

Whether you've been practicing, like my husband, since you were four years old (he grew up in a Transcendental Meditation community in Iowa), or you just close your eyes and go inward while riding the bus to work, you are meditating. You can think of meditation as time alone, relaxing your brain, or calming your thoughts so that you're not being pulled every which way.

If you feel like you don't have time to meditate, the basic *nugget* of meditation—the focusing or calming of the mind—is available to everyone in small increments at random moments of the day. By doing a mini-meditation, you can train your nervous system to rev down. I really like mindfulness meditation (based on an older form called vipassana, meaning "insight"). It's totally unreligious, un-culty, and immensely practical.

Here's a little taste:

Set a timer for five minutes.

Get into a comfortable, seated position.

Close your eyes, and bring your awareness to your breath.

Just notice the expansion and contraction of your belly. Observe your breath. Hang out with it.

FYI: Your attention won't settle for *long* on your breath—or anything else, for that matter. Our minds love to dart around and relive the past, fantasize about the future, and just generally do everything *but* settle down. As long as you're alive, your mind will never stop. It may melt into moments of thoughtlessness, but our mind's default mode is to bounce and bubble. One of the purposes of meditation is to help you experience a softer, slower bounce. By continually refocusing on the breath, the mind will decelerate a bit, landing on a second or two of peace; then it will wander again and will need to be refocused again!

That's okay. That's totally normal.

So whenever you notice your attention has wandered, bring it gently back to the breath, even if only for a few seconds. And when it wanders again, bring it back. Be gentle, and let go of judgment.

By the time your five minutes are up, you will have slowed down your mind (and your brain waves), making some space between thoughts: space for peace; space to receive; space to enjoy the present moment. You will find that your slowed-down mind—and connection to your breath—improves your whole day.

Almost every type of meditation practice, no matter the religion or philosophy, uses these basic elements of focus and breath

TO EACH HER OWN

There are many different types of meditation. Some involve repeating a mantra in the mind; others emphasize developing heightened awareness in the body. Some people begin by reading some spiritual literature and then meditate deeply on its meaning. As long as the mind is being focused—again and again— it's a form of meditation.

And no one does it perfectly. For instance, when I take a moment to try to calm my thoughts, I think of all of the things I need to do, or I start getting ideas for the script I'm writing or something I want to share in this book! And then, right after the thought comes up, I think, *Oh, that's a good idea. I'll remember that.*

Right.

And because I have so much on my mind, of course I end up forgetting it! So I've developed a little meditation workaround: When I'm trying to relax my mind with my eyes closed, I will open them again—just for a moment—to write something down on a pad I keep next to me. (I don't like making these notes on the phone, because it's too easy to get distracted by e-mails and texts.) Once I write down the idea or tidbit or to-do, I'll re-close my eyes and refocus. I try not to do it often, but my point is that it can be hard to just sit and have nothing important pop into your head. And I'd rather spend that time relaxing my mind than trying to engrain the tidbit into my memory.

So, discover what works best for you. A meditation practice is very personal, and yours may change over time.

as a technique for revving *down*. After you've gotten used to doing five minutes, feel free to do more.

Meditation is especially helpful when I know I'm heading into a crazy day, and I make sure I do it before going to work. I try to do ten minutes every morning, and when I can, I go for twenty. Beyond reducing my stress, I feel like it keeps me open to new ideas and possibilities.

SURRENDERING TO SLEEP

Obviously, there are periods in one's parenting life when sleep simply goes haywire: when babies are born, kids are sick, or the busyness of work and family life starts stealing precious *z*'s from your life. And when stress makes the body release cortisol, it causes an intense state of alertness. Because, as a mom, I've become a much lighter sleeper, I shoot upright in bed—in the middle of the night—at the sound of a loud noise from the street. My husband and I joke that I'm "meerkatting," like the little animal who stands erect when she hears a rustle in the grass. (We watch a lot of nature shows.)

So, yeah, sleep gets weird.

But we mothers can also get too familiar with our sleeplessness and begin to believe we don't need as much rest as we actually do. We pride ourselves on our five-hour nights and sleep-brag to our girlfriends, who have their own maternal Medals of Eternal Awakeness. Instead of closing our tired eyes, we space out on the computer or pour that extra glass of wine, which I get—*trust*— but when we make those choices too regularly, we can become sleep deprived.

And that's not good. Or cool. Not getting enough sleep depresses our immune function, messes with cognition, and hinders our body's ability to repair itself. In studies done on animals, total sleep deprivation caused them to lose all immune function and die within a matter of weeks.[7]

What constitutes sleep deprivation for us humans, exactly? There are conflicting views on how much sleep the average adult needs, and many experts argue for seven to nine hours, but let's put it this way: *You* need what *you* need to feel refreshed and energized, primed for a day of maternal adventures. I know for me, I do best on seven and a half hours. Seven is pushing it, and if I get less than that, I don't usually have a great day.

You may need to do some experimenting to figure out what your optimal sleep time is. So here are my suggestions:

MAKE A SLEEP DATE

One night a week, give yourself the bedtime of a fifth grader. Go to bed at eight or nine, without any digital technology, and just read a book. Give yourself permission to sleep those extra hours or to just loll around in bed.

If you don't fall asleep early or quickly, don't worry about it. Your body will be resting, and you will be sending it the message that rest is necessary and that you're allowed to get some. If you do this once a week, your body will begin to show you what it really needs.

When I take my sleep seriously and really try to recuperate from the stress of daily work, parenting, and wife-ing, I do a few things:

- I find that when I lay off sugar for a couple of hours before bed, I sleep better. This includes wine.

- I take an Epsom salts bath before bed. This relaxes me and gets me into sleep mode.

- On occasion, I have taken calcium magnesium. If your doctor approves, try 5-HTP (natural tryptophan).

SLEEP SCHEDULES

For newer mothers, I recommend that you get your baby on a sleep schedule as soon as possible.

I wish we had.

We were pretty lenient with Ella's sleep schedule for the first six or seven months. I couldn't bear to hear her crying, so my husband and I were still up at all hours of the night tending to her, making sure she was okay, taking turns on who would lose sleep.

When I told a close friend that we hadn't sleep trained Ella yet, she related her own story. She could not get her own child to sleep through the night, and she was becoming really exhausted, so she asked for advice from other moms on a mother-centric Facebook page she was a part of. She mentioned that if her daughter cried after being put to bed, she would go into the nursery and soothe her.

Expecting empathy, she got this instead:

YOU ARE F#*KING UP SO HARD followed by five hand-clapping emoticons. The commenter then instructed my friend to *put your baby down, put in earplugs, and drink a glass of wine.*

Although this was not professional advice from a doctor, my friend was sleep-deprived enough to get the hint, and soon her baby was sleeping, well, like a *baby.*

Another friend gave us a book entitled *Twelve Hours' Sleep by Twelve Weeks Old.* Although we were well past twelve weeks with Ella, we decided that enough was enough. Delirious from sleep deprivation, we got extremely serious about sleep training.

Of course, everyone has different beliefs about sleep training and letting babies "cry it out," etc., so you need to do what feels right for you and your children. But for us, when we got Ella on a schedule, and she adjusted, it was a Game Changer.

When Ella began sleeping through the night, that meant we could, too. I would still pop up like a meerkat in bed at any noise I heard, but if our busy New York street happened to be not so noisy that night, we were able to finally get some z's.

And, when I could finally predict her daytime naps, it freed me up to know what to expect; I knew when I could squeeze in a workout, get a little work done, prep dinner, clean, or even rest myself.

Thank goodness for sleep!

- I wear earplugs. I like Mack's. They have a slim fit, and they expand in your ear and really help mute exterior noise.

- I ask my partner to watch the monitor (Ella's a toddler, so we still have one) so I can sleep more deeply, without the pressure to get up in the middle of the night.

- I keep our bedroom dark. Our bodies are naturally stimulated by daylight, so bedrooms getting too much light from the street—or from our gadgets—can be difficult places to relax. The body's natural sleep hormone, melatonin, is triggered as the sun sets and darkness falls.

Once you get some good sleep, really try to see how you feel the next day. Are you brighter? More aware? Feeling like you want to be more productive? Those are signs, for me, that I got enough sleep. What are yours?

EXERCISE

Exercise reduces stress. *Especially* cardiovascular activity that causes you to break a sweat. Exercise boosts endorphins in the brain and calms the mind.[8] It can even improve your sex life. If you don't have time to get to the gym, find a ten-minute cardio workout video on YouTube to get your heart pumping. Just doing a little heavy breathing will get your happy neurotransmitters going and reduce your overall stress. We will expand on exercise in chapter 9.

CONSIDERING YOUR CAFFEINE CONSUMPTION

Although I don't plan to give up my coffee moonshine anytime soon, it's well documented that caffeine can increase feelings of stress and anxiety. By stimulating the adrenal glands, a dose of caffeine can give us what feels like fantastic energy, only to be followed by low blood sugar, irritability, and even anxiety for some users.

Scientists have recently discovered that caffeine sensitivity is determined by our genes,[9] with the vast majority of people having what is called "normal" sensitivity to caffeine, while others experience either high or low sensitivity. So even though your girlfriend can fall asleep after tossing back an espresso at 9:00 p.m., that same shot might keep you up all night scrolling frantically through Instagram. So listen to your own body and experience, rather than comparing yourself to others.

If you sense that caffeine might be exacerbating your stress, I encourage you to experiment with it. You can:

- Reduce your overall intake by half. There's a big difference between four cups of Joe a day and two. Or six and three. By dialing back, you'll start to get a sense of how the caffeine is affecting you.

- Stop at noon. Lots of people live by this rule. Caffeine's half-life is about four to six hours, so your noon cup has pretty much cleared your system between eight and midnight, right when you'd like to be asleep.

- Switch to green tea. Not only does green tea have less caffeine than coffee, but it's also simply a softer ride on your body and mind. It will still give you a morning perk and an afternoon bump, but it won't come with the same stress. You could also have coffee in the a.m. and switch to green tea for the afternoon, which I've done many times when I need a boost but am trying to cut down on caffeine.

- Switch to decaf. Either you can start mixing decaf and regular if you're ratcheting down, or you can make the leap into a decaffeinated existence altogether. If you choose to eliminate caffeine, be prepared to experience some withdrawal symptoms, like fatigue and headaches. They generally pass within a week or so, after which you should sleep like a baby and generally feel less stress.

With so many responsibilities tied to the schedules of others, many moms find they rely on caffeine—at least some of the time— and I relate. But keep in mind that quantity and quality matter. Check in with your internal stress level to figure out what works best for you.

SHARING YOUR TRUTH

We are all different. What stresses one mother out is a breeze for another, and vice versa, so you need to start understanding which thoughts, situations, and relationships raise *your* blood pressure. You can only start to manage your own stress level when you identify what, specifically, gets you worked up.

I have suffered with OCD and obsessive thoughts since I was a little girl. I used to have to touch the wall a certain number of times with a particular finger, in a certain way, or else I felt something terrible would happen to my family. I also had a bedtime routine that required me to look around the bed in a certain way, a certain number of times, before I could go to sleep, or else spiders would crawl on me while I slept (or some equally scary thing would happen). Thankfully, as I got older, these kinds of fears and thoughts got much better and even disappeared for about ten years.

But once I got pregnant, the scary thoughts began to creep back in. Will my baby be healthy? If I didn't feel her kick as much as she had the day before, I thought, Is there something wrong? Will she have ten fingers and ten toes? And then, of course, came worries

SCARY THOUGHTS

After talking with a lot of moms and doing some research, I've realized that many of us wrestle with scary thoughts that aren't necessarily connected to OCD. It's as if parenthood switches on a frightening new channel in the brain, conjuring stuff like: What if my kid falls out a window? What if the nanny steals my son? What if I drop my baby while I'm nursing? These and other scary thoughts can bubble up into the mind of the average mother, seemingly out of nowhere. Apparently, they're really common.

Obviously, these mental images can be a source of stress to any parent, but such scary thoughts tend to eventually dissipate. Sure, they may be replaced by other frightening thoughts more pertinent to your child's stage of development, but those should pass, too.

Some researchers believe that intrusive, scary thoughts in the minds of new moms are due, in part, to the tremendous hormonal flux that takes place in the postpartum period. Some other experts believe they may be a function of a parent's brain sort of figuring out the parameters of what's safe and what's not, in a time of intense stress and rapid neurological rearrangement. And although the intensity of

the thoughts tends to wane after infancy, protective thinking—based in some degree of fear—never really goes away for any parent.

Nasiba Adilova is a mother of three and the founder of the Tot (thetot. com), a curated, one-stop shop for conscientious parents that focuses on clean, nontoxic products. Originally from Russia, she lives with her family in Dallas, and she wrestled with her own anxious thinking when she became a mom. "In the very beginning, I was so paranoid about every little thing—even carrying my baby, I was, like, 'What if I slip and fall?' or, 'What if I run into a wall?' It was this feeling of fear and having to protect my baby, that instinct, that crazy instinct . . . an *animal* instinct on some other level . . . I'd never felt that before. I think it's a real, human, basic instinct that you have no control over."

I sure don't.

Understanding that scary thoughts are common—in fact, almost universal—can be very helpful to parents who are suddenly freaked out by the horror movies produced by their own minds. It was extremely comforting for me when I discovered that entire books had been written on the subject; I didn't feel so strange or afraid of my own brain.

about when she'd get older: Would she be bullied at school? Would she get hurt?

When Ella was actually born, my OCD got even worse. I just figured it was a dimension of the postpartum fear and anxiety I had as a first-time mom. I had scary thoughts about dropping her by accident or by falling asleep while feeding her because I was so tired. As she got older and sturdier, it really helped with my scary thoughts and OCD. Her stability in the world made *me* feel more stable. Talking to my husband was useful, too. I would tell him about specific fears I had, and just voicing them to someone I trusted helped a lot.

When I talk to someone new about the OCD, I make sure to preface the conversation with "I am going to share something with you that makes me feel very vulnerable, so I need you to support me." Once they've taken that on board, the conversation can be productive for both parties. Writing about it and sharing it with *you* helps me, too. It reduces the intensity and any shame that can accrue around it.

I may continue to wrestle with OCD for a long time to come. I'm trying to get a handle on it and am researching the best tactics for doing so, but in the meantime, I'm honest about it, and I do my best. When I talk to someone about it, it helps. And it also turns out to be a great way of lowering stress.

Here are our tools for reducing stress:

- Connecting with nature

- Learning to breathe

- Connecting with a friend

- Grounding yourself

- Meditation

- Surrendering to sleep

- Exercise

- Considering your caffeine consumption

- Sharing your truth

By using some of these tools, you will be able to slip more easily into the parasympathetic nervous system. Using them on a regular basis can prevent higher stress levels, allowing you to enjoy life more.

QUESTIONS TO CONSIDER

- Which situations in your life produce the most stress?

- Which anti-stress tool or tools are you most attracted to?

- Can you apply one of them this week? How about three times?

CHAPTER 6

Motherhood Around the World

HOW OTHER CULTURES DO IT

As a teenager, I lived in Italy and France for a while. I will always be grateful for that opportunity to broaden my horizons at such a young age. I loved exploring Paris and Milan and was fascinated by the delicious foods, the bold styles, and refreshing European attitudes. I even did my best to pick up the native tongues.

By living in foreign countries, I began to see things from a different angle. I became more aware of the invisible set of norms and standards I had grown up with, even in an unconventional household like mine. By leaving home, I not only came to appreciate what I'd received growing up in America, but I also opened up to a world of possibilities.

Vive la différence!

This chapter is my way of looking at motherhood through a wider lens. It wasn't until I'd had Ella that I realized I was behaving according to some invisible norms that simply seep into us as members of any society. They're neither good nor bad, but they're definitely there, so why not open up our perspective and see things in a new way? Let's look around and check out what the rest of the world is up to.

But first, here's an example of what I did.

The day I gave birth to Ella was the first day of production of season six of *Orange Is the New Black*. The writers wrote my character out of the first three episodes so I could be at home with my baby for six weeks, but after that it was "The show must go on!" as they say, and I was back at work.

When I returned to the set, it was very hard to be away from Ella. She was my first child, I had no idea what I was doing, and all of the amazing, terrifying learning curves that we talked about in the chapters on stress and control? I was smack-dab in the middle of them. I was in a bit of a daze, and I barely remember being on set during that time. If one more person had come up to me and joked, "Are you getting any sleep?" I might have decked them.

When my episode to direct came up on the schedule, Ella was just sixteen weeks old. I had had the opportunity to direct my first episode of *OITNB* during my pregnancy, and this, with Ella an infant, would be my second. When the producers asked if I felt I would be up for it, I blurted out, "Of course!" In fact, I was almost offended at having been asked. Sure, I'd just had a

> **With my newfound Mommy superpowers, I now look forward to how I will do things differently the next time.**

baby, but *obviously* I could helm the show and—just you wait—it'd be great!

I don't know why I felt I had something to prove.

So I did what any working mother would do: I made sure Ella would be well taken care of, packed up my breast pump, and sat my leaky boobs down in the director's chair. We worked long hours—often fifteen and sometimes as many as eighteen per day. And as the director, I was there before the crew arrived, and I never left until the very end of the day. Although directing is a true love of mine, man, I missed my baby. Every cell of my body was aching for her.

To manage the discomfort, I told myself my daughter would be proud if she understood what I was doing. And I tried to take Mila's words to heart and stay positive about work, never looking at it as a negative.

But when my milk started drying up from the stress of filming, and I realized that I was missing so much precious time of Ella's infancy, I found myself asking: Is this some kind of badge of honor that I'm wearing? Should I have fought for a longer maternity leave? Why is my saying, "I went back to work at six weeks after having a baby," making me so proud of myself? It was almost a macho approach to maternity. After all was said and done, I had to ask: What's so wrong with a four-month maternity leave so I can drink soup, heal, and bond with my baby?

With my newfound Mommy superpowers, I now look forward to how I will do things differently the next time. I hope to open up the choices for myself so I can stray a little from my "Laura can handle everything!" mode.

I was not the only one with this Momaholic approach to mothering. We seem to be convinced, at least in this country, that we are supposed to have it all, do it all, not to mention get our pre-baby bodies back in, like, five seconds. Why do we do this? And must it continue? Does every society have this pressurized approach to motherhood? What can we learn when we take a look around at other cultures?

The United States is wonderful in many ways, but we're not fantastic with supporting new moms during the postpartum period. Most other Western countries carve out plenty of time and space for a lying-in period (and beyond), whether staying in bed actually occurs or not. For instance, in Finland, a woman can leave her job a full seven weeks *before* her estimated due date and follow it up with sixteen more weeks postpartum—fully paid.

Canada, too, has a generous maternity package for its new mothers (paying 55 percent of one's previous income for twelve months or 33 percent for *eighteen* months), and many countries now include some kind of paternity leave so that both new parents can have time to relax and bond with baby.

Most Asian countries still respect a lying-in period for mothers. In India, special drinks designed to increase milk supply and lift hemoglobin levels are served to the new mother during the postpartum period.

In China, the average new mom stays at home—and mostly in bed—for one month after giving birth, during what's known as *zuo yue zi*, or "sitting the month" period. She is cooked special foods by her in-laws and encouraged to rest and recover. If she has no family to perform this role, China has "confinement centers" (which sound scary but are like hotels for new moms) designed to support her through this postpartum time. And if she has a job, she *also* gets a juicy maternity package. The point of *zuo yue zi* is to give a new mother time to relax, restore her strength, and bond with her baby.

In Latin America, the postpartum confinement, *la cuarentena*, lasts forty days and is a considered a special time for the new family to bond and adapt to parenthood.

So our American inclination to get back to work as quickly as possible may be driven by financial pressure (moms need their paychecks!), but it may also reflect gender issues, the ego's need to prove itself, or a certain American attitude about child-rearing.

It seems like, when it comes to parenting, Americans have entered the Age of Anxiety. We look to the media, or mommy blogs, in the belief that somehow the newest trend or philosophy can out-smart 200,000 years of Homo sapiens' progress.

I experienced an example of this just recently. I'd had a terrible night's sleep because our baby monitor illuminates our entire room every time Ella moves, let alone makes a noise. Well, my mother-in-law was visiting, and when I told her how poorly I'd slept and why, she said, "I never had one of those," eyeing the monitor sideways. "I'm going to throw that f#*king thing in the garbage."

I laughed.

Then she dropped some old-school mama wisdom on me: "You'll *know* something is wrong with your baby before that monitor lights up the whole room."

Ah, wisdom.

My friend Nicole, the survivalist, has worked for years with a tribe called the San (or Bushmen) in the Kalahari Desert of Botswana, and she's seen an entirely different way of raising kids. "As your children grow older," she says, referring to traditions among San families, "you're not expected to discipline them, and you're not expected to teach them."

What?

"Ever."

"Can you imagine if your only job was to love your children? That's it! Everything else is off your shoulders! You don't have to discipline your kids. Their aunties and uncles and grandmas and grandpas do that. They do something wrong? You don't say a word.

Someone else is on it. They need to be taught something? You don't do a thing. Someone else is on it. But you *are* expected to teach *other* people's kids."

When Nicole asked the San elders why they parent this way, she loved what they told her. "'So our kids will love us in our old age and take care of us!'" She laughs, bringing Kalahari sunshine right into the room.

"What a great thing, right? Because their only job is to *love their children.*"

Many Native American tribes also tend to raise children within broader, extended families and with an emphasis on noninterference. Whereas children in American society are viewed as the responsibility of the parent, or even sometimes as their parents' "property," in many Native homes, children are seen as autonomous individuals and given more decision-making freedom. Lessons are often transmitted through contact with nature and natural metaphors, and the child is guided by the community as a whole and not just by the nuclear family.

Having spent that time in Europe, I have always been fascinated by how women on the Continent approach motherhood. Whereas in the United States, once a baby is born, the parents bend their lives around the little one, in France, children grow up in their parents' world.

In her wonderful book *Bringing Up Bébé: One American Mother Discovers the Wisdom of French Parenting*, Pamela Druckerman, an American raising her kids in Paris, describes the differences she's noticed between American and French parenting styles. Baffled by French kids eating quietly—and *politely*—out at a restaurant, she discovered that built into the collective parenting ethos in France is the willingness to let children learn to wait—whether it's five minutes after waking up in the crib or for their designated snack time—just a little, every day.

These tiny pauses have immense benefits: Children learn tolerance of frustration, patience, resilience, confidence, and the recognition that they function in a larger constellation of people, all of whom have needs as well. And because French sleep-training habits and mealtimes are so universally accepted, parents don't waste time or energy trying to reinvent the wheel. *Oui, bien sûr*, each child is unique and must be cherished as such, but to the French, that doesn't mean she can't wait ten minutes for a snack!

French attitudes toward mothers are different, too. Pregnancy is seen as sexy, and women are encouraged to maintain their *femme* along with their *maman*. Writes Druckerman: "French pregnancy magazines don't just mention that it's okay to have sex. They spell out exactly how to do it—including lists of pregnancy-safe toys (nothing with batteries), aphrodisiacs (mustard, cinnamon, and chocolate), and detailed instructions on how to maneuver into third-trimester positions."[1]

Ooh la la!

Daphne Oz noticed cultural differences when she was pregnant with her first baby and on a trip to Italy. "I remember going to a beach and seeing these Italian mothers who were all lithe and healthy-looking—not like fitness freaks, just like they'd taken care of themselves."

I know exactly what she means: that cool, European look.

"And their beautiful children were all scampering around, going in and out of the water—and the kids couldn't have been more than three—and inevitably, once every twenty minutes or so, they would come running over for the moms to sort out some problem."

Every twenty minutes? I like *that* rate.

"And the moms would help if they had to but encouraged the kids to figure it out among themselves, and they would sit there and have their espressos and just enjoy each other's company."

La dolce vita!

"And I remember, in that moment, thinking: These women have brought children into *their* lives. They haven't completely reoriented themselves as something 'other.' And they are sexy, and they look smart and fun and engaged—and are still great moms! I have, as much as possible, tried to create that in our family," says Daphne. "We have our kids come into *our* lives and have our kids do things that we love to do and try to make sure that [our] zest for living stays alive."

I think she's really on to something here. And it seems there's wisdom to be picked up from many cultures. In the Netherlands, kids are encouraged to ride bikes in the rain to develop resilience and grit, and after about the age of four, they make their own lunch (from stuff Mom puts out). In fact, the Dutch approach to parenting looks like almost the opposite of our American model, with much less emphasis on things, overprotection, and striving for perfection and a refreshing focus on rest, routine, resilience, and family time.

In Spain, children stay up past 10:00 P.M. so they can participate in the fun and discussions over long family dinners. And when asked by an interviewer about whether raising her three kids was stressful, a Mayan mother in Mexico didn't understand the question; there was literally no word in her native language for "stressful," especially as it pertained to motherhood.[2]

I realize that I live in America, and my children will need to adapt to this culture, complete with its ups and downs. But looking at other countries always reminds me that there's no single route to happiness, that families can find their own "styles" (just like mine did, growing up), and guess what? We survive. And by looking at other ways of parenting, I'm reminded that motherhood can't be learned like math. There's no final answer on a blog somewhere, no perfection that can be reached. Motherhood is a million different experiences to be enjoyed, integrated, and grown into. We learn from all of those experiences: our highs, our lows, the daily routines, and sharing the journey with one another, no matter where we're from.

QUESTIONS TO CONSIDER

- What are some of the norms you've picked up from the society or people around you that might be good to question?

- Do you have any models of other mothers who are doing things differently? If so, what are they doing?

- Have you witnessed family life in other cultures? If so, what did you learn from that?

- Which other mothering techniques might you want to experiment with?

- How has this chapter helped you to identify elements of your own unique mothering style? How can you celebrate them?

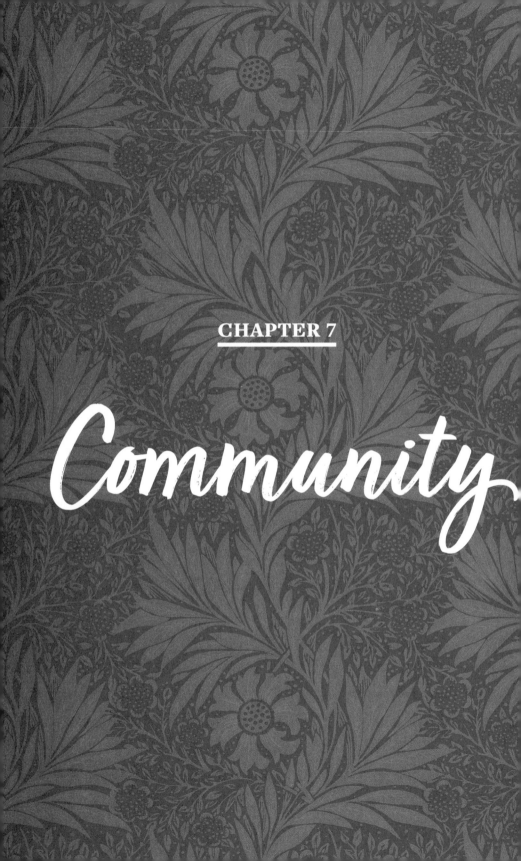

CHAPTER 7

Community

THE IMPORTANCE OF
A MOM SQUAD

For most of my life, I have been surrounded by people. As the youngest of five children, I was born into a mini-tribe, and we always had friends or exchange students from other countries staying over, too. Our home was so packed that my mother was once accused of running a halfway house!

The work I do involves hundreds of individuals working together in order to create something. The set of a TV show buzzes with energy and camaraderie; everyone has a role, and we all need one another to get an episode made.

And when I first got established in Los Angeles, I developed a great group of friends, and we'd get together often. I'd cook and entertain, and everyone felt right at home.

So, yeah, I'm used to having a community.

However, right before Ella was born, my husband and I moved our lives from LA to the East Coast. I had spent a lot of time there because I grew up in New Jersey, and *Orange* was shot in Queens, but after I left home at a young age, I never intended to move back east full-time. While working in New York, I rarely went out, except for the occasional outing with a fellow cast member (which was great), but I didn't have a community; most of my Mom Squad lived back in California, and of all the things I missed from my LA life, getting together with them was at the top of the list.

I tried to avoid my ache for my friends, and I lived in a certain amount of denial for a while. I mean, hey, I had my partner, and we were building our family, which I'd wanted my whole life, so what was the problem?

But when Ella was almost two years old, Ben went away to shoot two movies, back-to-back, in Eastern Europe. Living on the East Coast meant we were that much closer for stealing visits with each other, but it was during Ben's absence that my lack of a local community really began to dawn on me.

I would FaceTime with friends back in LA, and although screen-to-screen communication would suffice, nothing compared to getting together with a friend in real life.

But I was fine! Right?

The truth was, I was struggling with the adjustment to the East Coast. Sometimes I even resented our decision to live there, and I would blame Ben for making us leave our lives back in LA. But that wasn't true, and I was being unfair. We had made the decision together and I was simply wrestling with my grief. As my mother always taught me, I am responsible for my decisions, but I wasn't owning them, and that wasn't cool.

It was then that I decided to really build a life here. And that included community.

But how?

I was invited to a dinner; it would be a group of working moms getting together to talk about motherhood—what they loved about it as well as their struggles. It seemed like a safe place to break bread, have a glass of wine, and share.

My first instinct was to say no. I didn't need that! I only knew the women throwing it and just barely. But after getting a pep talk from my husband—still filming in Europe—I decided to go.

Suddenly feeling shy, I walked in tentatively. The party was in a beautifully lit room with a dining table in the center, elegantly laid. Candles flickered, and glasses of wine and champagne were being handed out. Luckily, one of the women I knew saw me right away and waved me over.

About thirty women mingled in the room. I was introduced to three of them, all working mothers in various interesting industries. The first woman I spoke to had a daughter Ella's age, and although the others' children were much older, everyone had a sense of empathy for what we were all going through, and it felt nice to open up with them.

After a moment we all sat down, and over dinner, we all shared about ourselves and about how motherhood had affected us: the good, the better, and the downright difficult. The stories ran the gamut from guilt, to lost intimacy with partners, to struggling with lack of sleep, aging, etc. To hear and share these stories was deeply profound for me. I felt community again. And I realized how very badly I had been missing it.

Every woman I spoke to for this book stressed how much community meant to her as a mother. Although the adage "It takes a village to raise a child" has become a cliché, that's because it's true. The more we lean on one another, the easier we make this experience, the better we feel, and the more stimuli we expose our kids to.

So I've been on a mission to build my Mom Squad: New York Edition. I've been trying to meet women—friends of friends, moms of Ella's playmates—and figure out if we have "friend" chemistry.

Which can be *awkward*.

It can feel like a blind date. Do we have coffee? Do we get a cocktail? A meal? What if it goes horribly wrong—do I have to stay through dessert? Can I say I have to let the babysitter go and get out of there? The whole thing reminds me of horrible online dating stories friends back home have told me about.

But I'm really trying. And there's no forcing these things. I find that chemistry between girlfriends is as elusive and wonderful as it is between partners. It takes a lot not only to support one another in momhood but also to have fun while we do it.

If you already have a thriving, supportive community around you, this chapter may help you see what it's doing for you on a deeper—even chemical—level. If, like me, you're trying to build community, this chapter should help you realize why it's important to have support beyond just your partner's. If you have a hard time reaching out or feel like you don't deserve help, I hope you come away from this chapter with tools and insights that will get your own Mom Squad started.

Let's start with community and the role it plays in us biologically.

We talked about oxytocin in an earlier chapter and how it makes you fall head over heels (to the point of obsession) with your children. Well, it was working on behalf of your relationships long before you became a mother, and especially in one important area: your friendships. And when that friendship is with a woman, there's even more oxytocin going around.

It's no accident that teenage girls hang around in giggling groups, and, when they're not together physically, they're talking and texting with one another ad nauseam. The female brain experiences massive surges in both estrogen and progesterone starting around puberty, and that estrogen increases the production of both oxytocin and dopamine (a feel-good neurotransmitter).

This surplus of oxytocin causes us to crave connection, and, because dopamine flows along with the oxytocin, when we do connect, we get immense *pleasure* from it. So that warm, relaxed glow you feel after a long call with a good friend? Besides the obvious benefits of connecting with a loved one, that call has also delivered a heady mix of oxytocin and dopamine—a real chemical payoff. In fact, Louann Brizendine writes in *The Female Brain*, "Connecting through talking activates the pleasure centers in a girl's brain . . . it's the biggest, fattest neurological reward you can get outside of an orgasm."

So long before we become mothers, we enjoy our girl tribe in a deep and visceral way. But what about later, as grown women? Dr. Brizendine adds, "Many women find biological comfort in one another's company, and language is the glue that connects one female to another."[1] So, suffice it to say, community doesn't just make our lives easier, it gives us very real pleasure while reducing our stress level as we exhibit the tend-and-befriend response. Isn't it great to know that our desire to connect is biologically supported? That we are *supposed* to hang out and talk?

I love that.

And of course, connection isn't limited to women. For years, my community was made up of mostly guys. Back in my poker days, I would host game nights, and I was often the only woman at the table. I'd also host viewings of UFC fights, serve homemade noshes, and yell at the TV as my place filled up with guy friends. Some of them would come over to the house to hang out even if I wasn't home!

When I reached out to Daphne Oz on the topic of community, she had a lovely take on it: "As adults, there are only a few phases of life when you can make a lot of new friends, and I think motherhood is one of them. I have worked hard to curate a group of women whose motherhood styles I really admire—they're different types of mothers, but there's something about them as women that I love and respect."

She elaborates: "You want a place where you don't have to explain yourself . . . people who are in the same life-[phase] that you're in, the same cycle that you're in . . . and you can trade secrets and advice and the greatest product you've ever bought with one another, but you can also have conversations that have nothing to do with motherhood."

Staying in touch with your peeps can happen in many ways, but Nicole had a nice routine that kept her community going. "When I lived in Portland, I had an every-other-Wednesday potluck. I called it Nature Nexus. We did it for five years, and it was *huge*. People would show up at my house: kids, people of all ages, people from babies up through age eighty. A core [group] would be there every time, but other people would rotate through. I always had my fire going, so we could connect around it."

And of course, because Nicole studied the Bushmen, she appreciates what's *really* happening at her potlucks, beyond the food and the fire. "When you have a group meet over time, kids grow up together, kids negotiate with other kids. And there's something really important about having intergenerational folks together. I think sometimes we get so isolated with people in our own age bracket . . . but in our past, when we lived in these hunter-gatherer communities, [interacting with one another] was what we were hardwired to do; that's in our DNA, so that's what really makes us feel the best . . . It's like a reminder, our DNA goes, 'Yes!' It was beautiful in its simplicity."

DOES SOCIAL MEDIA COUNT AS COMMUNITY?

Yes and no.

I'm not here to rain on your Twitter parade, but according to recent studies, our social-media lives may, in fact, be making us lonelier and more depressed. When students at the University of Pennsylvania limited themselves to just ten minutes of Facebook, Instagram, and Snapchat per day for three weeks, they showed a significant reduction in loneliness and depression compared to a control group that used social media as they normally would. They also experienced lower levels of anxiety and FOMO (fear of missing out).[2]

Maybe it's all the comparing ourselves to others. I remember hearing the expression "compare and despair," meaning that it's easy to believe that our lives are not as exciting or fulfilling as someone else's. And that's dangerous, because not all of what we see on social media is even real.

As adults, we can navigate this kind of input more easily, because we know that people are curating their profiles, putting up only what they want others to see, and that it's rarely the whole story. But for kids, it's much harder. To them, the online world can appear to be the actual world.

But the drawback to the whole social-media thing may also come down to something even more basic: lack of human contact. As much as

it *seems* like we are connecting with close friends—or even thousands of people—through our screens, it turns out there are no substitutes for eye contact, the sound of a human voice, and the warm energy emitted from another body. So, sure, stay in touch with people online, but don't let digital interaction be a substitute for face time with them. *Real* face time.

Even texting doesn't measure up in the communication department. In an interesting study, researchers found that a group of girls who'd been through a stressful set of tasks secreted oxytocin and experienced reduced stress levels when talking on the phone with their mothers immediately after the tasks—but *not* when they texted with them.[3] Even if their phone calls with Mom weren't particularly positive or soothing, just the sound of their mothers' voices calmed them down.

We seem to have forgotten the power that exists in listening, giving and receiving empathy, laughing at a joke (without emojis), and experiencing the delight of another's presence, even if only on the phone. Between our chronic busyness and Silicon Valley's savvy, it's been stripped from many of our daily lives.

Let's take it back.

ASKING FOR HELP

This is a challenge for me. One of the mantras I picked up at a young age was "If you want something done right, do it yourself."

But that doesn't always work, especially for a new mother. In fact, going it alone in the mom department caused a lot of problems—not to mention stress—for me and my partner. And I've noticed that many women in my social-media community also struggle with asking for help and write to me about it all the time. Clearly this isn't just my problem—it's ours.

It definitely was for Mila. "It took me a long time to realize that asking for help doesn't equal weakness . . . We fall into, 'I'm going to prove to everybody that I can do it by myself.'"

And that makes a lot of sense, given that America loves the DIY approach for just about everything. In fact, when ranked by individualistic versus collectivistic tendencies, the United States is number two in the world (after Great Britain) in valuing individualism. Canada, Australia, New Zealand, and the Netherlands follow right behind.

Which is not a bad thing. Respecting individualism means that it is deeply woven into our social fabric to take ourselves, our feelings, and our ambitions seriously. I watched my mother respect her individuality, and I'm grateful that she modeled that for me. I would have neither an acting nor a directing career, let alone the opportunity to write this book, if I'd sunk back into the collective and waited for those around me to give me the thumbs-up.

So shouldn't I be able to bring my rugged individualism to the motherhood party?

I mean, sure, it's *possible* to keep an I-can-do-this-all-by-myself stance as a mom, but over the long haul, it's not good for me or Ella or the people around us. And it flies in the face of human history; running a family is, by its very nature, a collective enterprise. Anyone from a large family, or anyone who was nurtured by a larger community, can tell you that. But so many of us these days exist in nuclear families, out of daily reach of our extended tribes, and continue to function from those invisible norms inside of us, the ones that whisper, "You can do this *by yourself!*"

So if asking for help feels hard, there's a good reason; you, like many of us, may have been conditioned by society to go it alone. But now it's time to move in the other direction.

With nine kids to raise, Dee needed help from others just to get by. "Thank God I had an ex-mother-in-law who came in, because I did Broadway for years—with nine children—so it takes a village. You have to network with other parents, too. Sometimes you gotta go, 'Okay, I'm off this week, so I'll carpool for *you.*' It takes a lot, and you want to make sure your child is safe."

In Mila's case, her spouse cracked the code. "Ashton stopped asking me. He always knew I would say I didn't need help, so he just started *doing.*" She smiles with obvious gratitude. "That helped me a lot. He stopped asking me what I needed and just *did it.*"

ALLOPARENTING

If you're concerned about getting help or feel guilty about letting someone else care for your child, consider this: Humans are one of a handful of mammalian species that permit their children to be nurtured, or cared for, by other adults. These other caregivers are known as alloparents (literally "other parents"), and they can be family members, trusted hired help, or good friends. Some scientists believe that our willingness to allow alloparenting is one of the factors that sets humans apart from most of the animal kingdom and that by being exposed to more individuals in our "village," we developed language and bigger brains.[4]

Call the babysitter!

If you have trouble asking for help, practice with little things, like:
"It would really make my day a bit easier if you could . . ."
"I would so appreciate if you would . . ."
"Can you help me with . . . I would love to help you with something you need tomorrow."

If you still find it hard to ask for help, think of it this way: Your loved ones will get some oxytocin pleasure from helping you! Let them.

BUILDING YOUR MOM SQUAD

Being with people feels good; it's in our DNA to hang out together. So although it's great to get advice and vent our frustrations online, don't deny yourself the pleasure of some in-person bonding with friends. There are lots of ways of doing it. Here are some tips to get you started:

- Ask two of your closest girlfriends to each invite one mom-friend over. Bring a friend of your own, and suddenly three becomes six. This is an easy way to meet people who are all vouched for.

- Reach out to a small group on social media and ask them to come over for a potluck. With each mom bringing a different dish, there's very little work involved, and it's a great way to bring the digital world into the real world.

- Host a wine night, assigning different types of wine to a few moms, cheeses, etc., to the other ones. Voilà! Instant fun.

- Find a local chef you like, and invite some friends over for a cooking lesson. If you split the cost among a group of six or eight, the price can be really reasonable and the evening incredibly fun. You can also learn new culinary tricks to use at home.

- Set up a collective nature hike.

- Set up a stripper class for you and your friends, and learn some fun tricks to bring home to the bedroom.

- Amber's saucy suggestion: Throw a sex-toy party, considered the twenty-first-century Tupperware party. There are sites online to help you organize one. Get a sex educator to come over and teach you and your friends some fun things you can do with the newest toys.

Here are the tools we've discussed:

- Asking for help
- Building your Mom Squad

Community is key to our well-being. It's one of the reasons I wrote this book—to help us all connect with one another. By cultivating community, we have richer, more loving, and more connected lives.

QUESTIONS TO CONSIDER

- Is there a friend you haven't phoned in a while? Or gotten together with? What's stopping you from reaching out?
- Can you try asking for help at least once this week?
- What are you looking for in a Mom Squad? What can you contribute to one?
- Is there an event you can organize that would bring some people together on a regular basis? Is there a group that you could join?

CHAPTER 8

Keeping the Love Alive

TIPS FOR NURTURING
YOUR RELATIONSHIP

Every relationship is unique. Some are short, and others last a lifetime. Some are full of drama, while others seem to flow along with nary a ripple. The members of my Mom Squad come from all different types of relationships—of different durations and configurations. I've gone from a ten-year relationship to a three-year relationship to finally meeting my husband (whom I waited thirty-six years for!), and now we are parents.

For many couples, once kids are in the mix, taking care of the relationship that *produced* those kids seems like the first thing to slide. Life suddenly gets put on a schedule; sleep is interfered with; beloved offspring need protection, care, feeding, chauffeuring, and attention. This puts an obvious strain on the couple as the energy that was once directed at each other is now moving in a million new and important directions.

S ome couples never bounce back from this rearrangement. They enter the new status quo and just stay there. And I get it. It's not easy to put the brakes on the Kid Train and get back on the Couple Train. Doing so can require overcoming resistance, but we are committed to doing that. In fact, most of my friends, my siblings, and even doctors I know with kids—none of us want our relationships to stagnate.

Who does?

But very real issues can come up to sabotage a connection: Some couples struggle to communicate; others have a hard time navigating the physical changes that come with motherhood or with aging; many of us are just tired—soul-fatigued, as my husband calls it. For some couples, it's all of the above. And on top of everything else, we're all changing, all the time.

This chapter is chock-full of tools you can use to work on your relationship; some may be new to you, whereas others you know but maybe haven't picked up in a while. In fact, for this chapter, let's throw out the word "tools" and think of them as logs, because keeping the love alive is like stoking a fire, not letting it lose its heat, and saying, "Absolutely not" to its petering out. It's about declaring, "We are going to be here for our children no matter what, so let's make sure that we're here together."

Throw another log on the fire.

I faced the need to feed my relationship with Ben for the first time when Ella was just a few months old. Like most new moms, I felt really attached to my baby. My whole being—mentally, emotionally, and physically—was wrapped up in her, which was not a bad thing, per se.

I mean, hey, I'm her mother.

But after a while, it was becoming imbalanced and it was affecting us. I didn't like leaving the apartment, and I was struggling with postpartum anxiety. I knew I needed space and some breathing room, but I was too afraid to leave Ella.

"We need to go somewhere," Ben said one night while I folded baby clothes. "We need to be *us* again."

I immediately tensed at the idea. I couldn't leave our daughter. Even though I knew that Ben and I needed time alone, I couldn't be away from Ella. It felt way too soon.

Ben booked us a hotel room on the other side of town. He wanted to get us as far from our apartment as possible while remaining close enough to rush home if necessary. As a partner, I knew I was neglecting our relationship, so I finally agreed to go.

But the next night, when we entered the hotel room, I burst into tears.

"I have to be with Ella! I can't be here." I couldn't stop crying.

The stress I felt was intense and inexplicable. We'd left Ella in loving, competent hands, but I felt as though we needed to rush home that minute. My cells buzzed with anxiety. I was uncomfortable in my own skin. I felt angry. Angry with myself for not being able to be present with my partner, for feeling like I needed to rush back to our daughter. I was angry with Ben for making me leave her.

On top of everything else, we're all changing, all the time.

I tried to pick a fight so I could leave. I was desperate, but I wasn't sure why. I love Ben beyond comprehension, but Mama Bear was being poked in a way that made her want to hurt someone if I couldn't get back to my daughter. I was like a caged animal, pacing in the hotel room, staring at my husband with inexplicable resentment.

He approached me carefully and gave me a long hug. He wiped my tears. "I miss her, too," he said.

He then picked up the hotel phone and ordered us some dinner: two hamburgers and a big mess of fries. Although I was having a hard time getting into the spirit of our getaway, some greasy carbs would help. I started to thaw.

And some uninterrupted sex wouldn't hurt, either. Since having Ella, we'd become like teenagers with their parents in the next room—quiet and careful. To be able to throw caution out the window sounded amazing.

As the hours ticked by, I let myself relax and realign with my pre-motherhood world, the one in which my partner got my undivided attention, and I his. As soon as I gave myself permission to be off duty for the night, knowing that our daughter was with someone we trusted, Ben and I could find each other again.

In hindsight, our hotel mini-vacation seems like an obvious solution. However, when your kids need you, deprioritizing your *own* needs, and those of your partner, feels automatic. But in order to have a healthy relationship, it's important to find balance. So let's explore some ways to keep your love fire burning. The suggestions coming up are simple, fun, and will remind you both of what you have together.

GETTING OUT OF THE HOUSE

I realize now that our little getaway worked for a number of different reasons, but primarily, we'd gotten ourselves out of our own home. This may sound obvious, but it bears exploring. By leaving our own environment, we were not only leaving our baby, but all sorts of cues that produce stress in us. It's not until you get away that you realize that even a few dirty dishes in the sink can set your teeth on edge or that an unmade bed can make you feel bad about yourself. By getting away from all these subtle triggers, our bodies and minds had the chance to relax.

By leaving home, we'd also taken ourselves off the clock, at least for a while. Having an infant meant that life was run by Ella and her schedule: Nap time, mealtime, bath time, and bedtime had become our new masters, and our nervous systems had become obedient little soldiers, saluting the clock. Although this made for structure and stability for Ella, it was draining spontaneity from us. By getting off the baby clock (and kids, tweens, and teens have schedules, too), our nervous systems could relax into what felt like an endless and indulgent evening. That expansive feeling of timelessness was more delicious than the French fries!

Finally, Ella is always observing us both carefully, and I am constantly trying to model good behavior for her. I try to watch my language, I try to bring her positive energy, and I try to do my best when I'm around her. It feels like part of Nature's plan that we do our best to model positive behavior for our kids, but it's also a subtle responsibility that's great to drop every once in a while.

With all these pressures gone, we could rebel, let down our parent guards, and remember what we'd enjoyed about each other before Ella came along to grow us up. We could be honest about our fears, frustrations, and fantasies and even curse if we needed to. A familiar space reopened between us that had gotten cramped and tight. When we both saw that we were still there for each other and weren't just Ella's caretakers, our bond got stronger. And some of these things, we could only achieve away from home.

Members of my Mom Squad also prioritize taking time away from the kids to keep their love fueled.

Daphne: "I really make it a priority to have alone time with my husband, to listen to him, have him listen to me, to remind ourselves of all the ways we fell in love with each other. And all the ways that our relationship is so much richer and deeper now, post-kids. It's *evolved*. And how do you make sure you water that flower, too? It's not going to be the same easy, carefree experience of romance that you had before you had kids together, because it can't be. You're so much more vulnerable with that person *and* so much more secure in that relationship. It's infinity times more powerful, more bonded, deeper and richer . . . and I think you just have to find ways to access that."

Dee also manages to make the time and the space to care for her relationship. "I always made sure once a week we had a date night. It can be a movie or dinner or meeting up with friends, because sometimes, as a couple, you need to talk it out with someone else. I always made sure we went out with couples with children and talked about parenting."

She also recommends longer getaways. "And twice a year, just get away for a week. That kills you as a mother, because you never want to leave the child, but it's so important, because

BUDGET BONDING

This doesn't have to be expensive. Pack a picnic with a bottle of wine, bring some robes or comfy clothes, and flop into bed at a cheap motel near you. And if you want to spend even less, I have friends who swap homes with other friends for the weekend in order to shake things up. Kids go to Grandma's/Mom and Dad, and have a whole new apartment! The point is being *out* of your own environment and having some fun.

[you run the risk] of not being that spontaneous person . . . And it kills the relationship, because where's your bond?"

HAVING FUN TOGETHER

Do some of the things you did before you had kids. This will remind you of who you are as a couple. And now that you're more bonded—as parents—it may be even more fun!

When Ben and I first got together, one of our favorite pastimes was to hang out in a dive bar and play a card game called Rummy 500—a fun, adrenalized version of Rummy. We used to play together for hours, enjoying the competition, goading each other on.

Amber and her husband, David, have a similar ritual: "We play Crazy Eights, which is the most grandmotherly thing ever, but we used to play it all the time before Marlow. Talking s#*t, having drinks for hours."

Sometimes it's about creating *new* fun. Daphne and her husband like to keep it fresh. "[We] push each other all the time; [for instance] I want to see more live music this year, so we're going to do more of that, and he wants to travel a little bit more, so maybe once or twice a year we will take a trip away by ourselves to a place we wouldn't take the kids."

By doing new things, you will be continually introducing adrenaline into the mix, which can keep your relationship fun and exciting.

COMMUNICATION

Communicating, for me, is about putting myself on the line and sharing my personal perspective. And to do that, I have to be ready for disagreement, which can be scary. But it's by putting ourselves

GET HELP IF YOU NEED IT

Every partnership falls into its habits, some good, some bad. But familiarity often breeds contempt, and partners can get lazy, or afraid of deepening intimacy, and what began as a honeymoon becomes a painful and lonely experience.

I know many who have sought out counseling, from therapists, counselors, or friends, in order to support their relationships. I've even been asked to sit in as a mediator with married friends of mine who have been together for close to ten years, with two children. Whenever one would express a feeling about something, the other would get defensive and attack. And of course, that would provoke the person who'd spoken up to attack back, and before you know it, there was a big fight. Knowing this about themselves, they asked me to be a neutral person in the room. To just be present, so they felt safe to open up and not be attacked. So I did. And they were able to communicate.

Others I know have studied Nonviolent Communication

techniques, which help break down difficult conversations into specific parts: One partner reports to the other first what she observes, then what she feels, followed by stating her needs, and finally making a request of her partner. And vice versa.

Based on the idea that we can all operate from empathy and compassion—we just sometimes lack the tools to do so—Nonviolent Communication was developed by Marshall Rosenberg in the 1960s, while he worked with civil rights activists. I find the technique interesting, because it helps people distill potential conflicts down to their most basic and important parts—our feelings, needs, and desires—and offers techniques to help each partner feel truly seen and heard. And when it comes to relationships, what matters more than that?

At the end of the day, use whatever works. I am a firm believer in reaching out for help when it comes to the sticky, difficult issues of life. A good partnership is always worth working on.

on that line—coming to the communication table—that we get connected, whether there's agreement or not.

To love is to be vulnerable, and we find strength in exploring viewpoints different from our own. As a couple, we can evolve to find new agreements and understanding, but that evolution can only take place through communication.

And truly effective communication, as with everything else, takes work.

I know couples who have been together for years—decades, even—who simply don't communicate openly. But when important things aren't addressed, they don't just go away; they fester. Like a slow, creeping mold that you can't yet smell, the problem is growing, and it won't disappear.

This situation can lead individuals to simply end the relationship and never talk again. Although that doesn't mean the mold's gone away. Others may feel like, after a long while of not dealing with them, there are too many unaddressed issues in the relationship, and they don't even know where to start.

For me, being willing to be vulnerable is the first step. But my partner needs to make it safe for me to open up. If he doesn't make it safe, that's a major barrier to talking freely.

And we don't always have to be talking about the heavy stuff. Humor bonds people, too. When I asked Amber how her husband, David, helps her in his own unique way, she mentioned his humor: "David is maybe the only person who can pull me out of the darkness my mind can go to . . . with inappropriate humor. Some of the jokes he's made in the ten-plus years we've been together . . . if anyone else said that, I'd be, like, 'You're dead. I'll never talk to you again.'"

She smiles. "He will find the thing that makes me laugh, whether it's poking fun at me or the situation or something totally awful. The inappropriate humor that he and I connect on kind of draws me back into the present and takes me out of the headspace I'm in. And that's really special, and that's not something you can get from friendship. It's a special thing."

Nicole also has a great trick for bonding with her kids that can be used in any relationship. She makes a crackling fire, invites her sons to sit around it with her, and they watch what she calls "bush TV." While staring at the fire, even teenage boys begin to talk.

We sometimes forget that natural things like fires, sunsets, and oceans can engage us completely. Just walking or driving together past natural scenery can be relaxing. When our minds are focused externally in a soft and calming way, we settle into ourselves. Pretty soon, we just start expressing things that bubble up. This approach can be great for couples, especially when looking each other in the eye feels too intense or even confrontational.

LIMITING SCREEN TIME

This may sound like a no-brainer, but it can be hard to do. Statistics vary, but it's estimated that the average American checks her phone anywhere from 47 to 300 times a day! And when we do it in the presence of another human being, it can cause damage to that relationship by stirring up subtle feelings of rejection in the other person. Recent studies show that the phenomenon of "phubbing" (snubbing someone by picking up the phone—we've all done it and had it done to us!) has a negative impact on relationships, causing spouses to feel less marital satisfaction, and even depression.[1] The theory goes that being phubbed threatens four of our basic needs: belongingness, self-esteem, meaningful existence, and control. That may sound extreme, but pay attention to how you respond, on a subtle level, next time someone does it to you.

And no, being with someone while you're *both* on screens doesn't count. There are many times Ben and I will work next to each other on our devices, but we don't classify that as "time together." Because although we like working next to each other in the same space, at those times we aren't fully present. It's important to bond without devices between you.

Recently, Ben and I took a vacation—our first in two and a half years. I honestly didn't think I could do it; the last time we'd traveled as a family was very difficult for me. I felt like I couldn't create a reliable, stable environment for my child on the road, that I couldn't protect—or re-create—my family's ecosystem away from home. I struggled with this for close to two years, so our solution was just not to travel.

CONNECTION PROTECTION

"What did you do today?" It's a common question asked by family members around the world every day. And it's not a bad thing; on the contrary, it shows we care about the lives of those we love. But Nicole taught me that, by asking your partner or your kid what they've *done*, you are putting attention on productivity versus connectivity. Emphasizing productivity could just provoke a dull recital of a checklist.

Instead, she suggested asking things like "What happened today that made you laugh?" or "What made you happy today?" Those sorts of questions will bring your family member into a feeling-based mode of reflection and open them up in a whole different way. I do this consciously now, and it really makes a difference.

Try it!

But that wasn't sustainable. We finally realized we simply needed some time off—together—so we decided to go away as a couple. We would take the plunge and be away *two whole nights!* Which obviously doesn't seem long enough, and yet felt like it was too long. I'm a mom, so no decision about being away from my kid quite fits—just like those damn pajamas she keeps growing out of.

Nonetheless, we decided to go, and we promised each other: NO CELL PHONES.

We gave Ella's caregiver the number to the hotel and our room number, and we knew that if there was an emergency or she needed to contact us for any reason, someone would find us immediately. We also set specific times during the day to check in. Besides that, no screens were allowed: no cell phones, computers, iPads, nothing. We were committed to not having our devices on us for a full two and a half days. Our only forms of entertainment were one book each, our environment, and each other.

APPRECIATION

I hear again and again from the Mom Squad how important it is to keep appreciation going between partners. Whether it is a simple "Thank you" for a task done or a "You're beautiful" at an unexpected moment, words of appreciation seem to serve as real emotional glue between us, deepening our connections.

Mila's husband practices this all the time. "Ashton has always been amazing at showing appreciation, so whether it's 'Thanks for making this dinner,' or if I'm waking up every morning with the kids, he says, 'Thank you so much.' He's never gotten to a place in our relationship where he's complacent, or expectant of things. Having that little bit of 'I see you, I appreciate you, and I'm with you' is . . . everything."

Although it's easy over the long haul to get lazy about this stuff, the women I spoke to with long-term, happy marriages maintained a certain level of respect between partners that rarely wavered.

Little things go a long way. Whether it's a loving compliment, a word of encouragement, giving thanks, or offering a home-cooked meal, these gestures tend to soften and open the relationship. It can even be as simple as a note: a Post-it scribbled with a message and stuck under your partner's bathrobe hook as a little surprise after a shower; a Post-it in the bag taken to work; a short love letter hidden in a suitcase when he or she is leaving on a trip. These little things mean a lot and cost little or no money. What are some ways you can show appreciation to your partner?

It. Was. Fantastic.

We played in the ocean. We laughed and talked and laughed some more. We relaxed into places in ourselves that technology had sneakily crept into. Without our phones, dinner tasted better, our sleep got deeper, and our bond grew even stronger.

Obviously, smart phones are now a part of daily life, so this requires agreement and commitment. Lots of people start by simply declaring a phone-free dinner, agreeing to turn off technology for the duration of that meal every night. Maybe next, there's a no-phone-in-bed policy. Sure, let it be on a desk across the room, but let bed be a more restful, intimate space.

Do what you can and what works for your life. Everyone is different. But as Amber says so delicately: "GET OFF YOUR PHONE!"

HAVING SEX

One of the most basic, intimate forms of communication is sex. Sometimes talking leads to sex, and sometimes sex leads to talking, but either way, sex with a partner brings us closer; it creates intimacy.

I recently sat down with Jill Blakeway, the acupuncturist I mentioned earlier. Termed a "Fertility Goddess" by the *New York Times*, she is also the author of *Sex Again: Recharging Your Libido*. Jill has helped thousands of people dealing with sex, fertility, and relationship issues over the last two decades. A mother of a daughter in her twenties and married to her husband for more than twenty years, Jill is a fount of wisdom, and we had a lot to talk about. First, I asked her what can get in the way of couples having sex.

"I think we are very busy," she says in her pretty British accent. "I think Americans—and I include Western Europeans in this—we're extremely busy . . . and we're tired."

You can say *that* again.

"We are also bombarded with sexual imagery that is very unrealistic, and that's gotten worse . . . Internet porn and even magazines—you know how much Photoshopping gets done in your profession."

Yes, I do.

"That sets up very unrealistic expectations, and we internalize things about our bodies. Social [media] doesn't help . . . and all those Instagram models. But the truth is, your body changes quite a lot after being pregnant, and you need to allow it to. And not fight it."

I love that.

"Men are visual," she says, "so we have learned to be performative, sexually. We've sort of trained ourselves to do that. But in order to really let go and have an orgasm, you do have to learn to *not* be performative. Sex is one of our few experiences of oneness, energetic *oneness*. That feeling of oneness, that feeling of connection—that's going to refuel you better than just about anything to look after a little one."

So the fertility goddess is saying that sex improves parenting?

"But to do that you have to let go of your expectations about your body. If you're thinking, 'Oh, my God, is he looking at my stretch marks? Or my muffin top? Or the jiggly bit under my arm?' then you're not going to let go enough to enjoy sex. I think women, in order to orgasm particularly, have to let go of *self* a little bit. Men tell me all the time that they barely notice. And in a loving relationship your partner should be reinforcing how sexy you look. And kissing your tummy that isn't quite where it was is probably a good start."

Jill also points out, "Great sex doesn't always look like [what] happens in the movies. Great sex can sometimes be a quickie. Great sex can sometimes be quiet and intimate. Great sex can be all sorts

EXERCISE: RELEASING RESENTMENT

When we have resentments, we can get stuck. We start ruminating on them, doubling down on our hurt and the need to be right. Of course, the human ego likes to dig in, but that often flies in the face of our personal happiness; harboring a resentment will hurt *me* much more than the person I'm resenting, causing stress and tension and a string of negative thoughts. Who needs that?

Every relationship requires negotiation, and often we must meet the other person halfway. When things are difficult, relationships also require flexibility and forgiveness. It's best to release the resentment so you can have some true perspective on the problem. The issue may need some courageous attention, and being all pissed off won't make working it out any easier.

In her book *Energy Medicine*, Jill Blakeway teaches a form of breathing that she adapted to help others discharge resentment. It's simple, but it helps to let go of all the negativity you can carry around when you are feeling resentful.

Practice breathing in gently for a count of six and then breathing out smoothly, also for a count of six. Don't force it. By breathing gently and evenly, you will be balancing your sympathetic with your parasympathetic nervous systems. This will slow down your heart rate and bring you some calm. Once you're in the rhythm, imagine exhaling your resentment. You might see dark energy or heaviness or whatever tension you may be carrying leaving you. Just imagine it's getting blown away on your exhalations. Really give yourself permission to let it go.

With every inhalation, feel the cooling and expanding power of the fresh air. Let yourself be filled by it. After a few minutes, you will feel lighter and more open.

You may need to do this exercise a few times to let go of difficult feelings, but it will help start moving them out.

of ways, but it connects you energetically to your partner in a way that I think is really important. I wrote *Sex Again* because so many patients told me they stopped having sex with their partner, and I thought they were missing some energetic connection that is deeply bonding . . . and gets you through the tough times."

When I ask her why so many people stop having sex completely, she says, "It varies hugely. I often find resentment is at the bottom of it. Resentments build up. After having kids, couples tend to get less sleep, there's more stress, and you simply have a shorter fuse. Priorities shift, so, at times, you let fights linger. Handling problems and resentments just gets harder and takes too much energy that one doesn't have."

And the solution to resentment stopping sex?

"Sometimes the way out of resentment is to *have sex* and see your partner as vulnerable and connected and human and frail in some

OXYTOCIN, PART THREE: THE MAGIC OF TOUCH

Touch is powerful. Gentle, loving, skin-to-skin contact not only makes us feel good, but also bonds us with the person we're touching. And that's not just a conceptual thing. Touching, cuddling, or massaging someone we care about—lover or child—produces oxytocin, which deepens our primal connections with one another.

If your relationship is feeling a little stale, or there seems to be distance between you, ask yourself how much touching you've been doing lately. Although oxytocin is also secreted during sex (and lots of it!), you don't have to retreat to the bedroom to renew your connection. Simple tactile affection can build bridges, calm nerves, and bring you back to your original bond. Oxytocin has been shown to increase empathy and generosity and may be a factor in that energetic connection that Jill described.

ways . . . I think sex does that for us. I often encourage people to just start . . . just *do* it."*

Resentment can be hard to let go of. This is also something that outside help can assist in getting to the root of. As Jill describes it, "Resentment is really toxic, and you need to deal with it if you're going to do a journey with someone."

Boy, is that true.

I know that when I feel close to my partner, I am a better parent and all-around human. Jill continues, "It's important to make time for your relationship. Your relationship restores you, and that makes you a better parent. Being lonely and isolated in a marriage where you're resentful and shut down is not helping you be the best parent you can be."

LIVING YOUR COMMITMENT

During a wedding, a couple shares vows, which are a mutual code of ethics. Even unmarried partners have understandings and agreements between them. But we don't just express these ethics once and file them away for the rest of the relationship. We need to keep our commitments fresh and real. We need to let them penetrate our daily attitudes and behaviors. And, as we discussed in the chapter on control, one's attitude can affect everything.

Marcus Luttrell, author of *Lone Survivor*, once said, "You don't get to *keep* your trident (the pin you get when you are designated a SEAL); you earn it every day. Even when you retire, you have to represent the ethos, the behavior, and the responsibility of a Navy SEAL."

---

* If you're in an abusive relationship, having sex to build your bond might not be the right approach. If you need help, reach out to someone you trust, and there are multiple hotlines you can call.

I feel this beautifully applies to any kind of partnership. We earn our trident, our wedding band, or our agreement of commitment, however the agreement stands, every day.

So, let's throw another log on the fire.

Here are the tools we've discussed:

- Getting out of the house

- Having fun together

- Communication

- Limiting screen time

- Having sex

- Living your commitment

By using some (or all) of these tools, you'll be giving more energy to your relationship, inviting it to thrive and grow.

>>>>>>>>>>>>>>>>>>>>>>>>><<<<<<<<<<<<<<<<<<<<<<<<<<

QUESTIONS TO CONSIDER

- What is one way you can contribute to your relationship today?

- Is resentment starting to creep into your partnership? If so, how would you like to address that?

- How's your sex life? Are there issues between the sheets that need to be addressed?

- Can you list five things you appreciate about your partner?

>>>>>>>>>>>>>>>>>>>>>>>>><<<<<<<<<<<<<<<<<<<<<<<<<<

CHAPTER 9

Mama Needs Some TLC

THE BENEFITS OF SELF-CARE

I recently reached out to my social-media community and asked what they considered to be the toughest thing about motherhood that is *not* generally talked about. The consensus was overwhelming:

Mom guilt.

I couldn't believe how many comments I got about this particular topic. And although mom guilt tends to show up in just about every area of a mother's life, it's particularly strong around the subject of self-care. It seems like those two little words put together, "self" and "care," cause a vicious undertow of guilt in us. It's as if, as mothers, we all vie for some illusory trophy for self-sacrifice.

And it seems especially bad for mothers who work outside the home (even though staying at home with children can be just as hard or even harder). It's as if, after having spent a whole day away from our kids, the idea of then going to a salon or the gym or otherwise getting some Me-time becomes unacceptable.

But if we *don't* refuel our bodies, minds, and spirits, we not only start to lose our identities, but also have nothing left to give our families. Eventually, we become depleted. And although martyrdom is a solution for some people, it's not sustainable. So self-care is the furthest thing from an indulgence; it's a necessity.

Daphne puts it really well: "I've heard a lot of parents say, 'My life is on hold for twenty years until my kids don't need me anymore,' which is the most [messed-up] sentiment I've ever heard, for so many reasons: (a) because I hope my kids *never* don't need me, (b) because nobody's life can afford to be on hold for twenty years . . . you're guaranteed nothing."

Nothing.

"I feel like when we put that kind of pressure on ourselves and on our kids, we steal the joy out of what should essentially be part procreation, part the richest, most wonderful relationship you'll ever create, and that's with your kids and with your family."

I couldn't agree more.

Self-care doesn't have to be a tipsy long weekend away with friends (although those are fun). Self-care is simply bringing your attention back to yourself, your needs and desires, on a regular basis. We mothers don't tend to have huge chunks of time to ourselves, so self-care may come in slivers, but that's okay. It's about sending the message to your inner self that it's okay to slow down, to receive, and to be replenished. That message *alone* is a powerful thing.

> *Self-care is the furthest thing from an indulgence; it's a necessity.*

This is especially necessary for modern moms who don't live with extended family or have close relationships with neighbors.

When a woman's community is like an actual village, there can be—paradoxically—more time for self-care; a sister takes her kid for the afternoon, or her parents take the child for the night. A healthy community understands, and can support, the needs of the individuals within it.

But if, like me, you don't have family members at your fingertips, it falls upon us to make the very important decision to give to ourselves. And even enjoy it. Setting aside time for self-care is not always easy and won't ever be perfect, but I'm determined to practice it.

So can we agree to give mom guilt the ole heave-ho?

In previous chapters, we've put together a bunch of tools that can support your self-care:

- Asking for help

- Making clear choices

- Connecting with nature

- Meditation

- Surrendering to sleep

- Exercise

- Sharing your truth

- Calling a friend

- Nourishing your partnership

In this chapter, I hope my Mom Squad and I will inspire you to take self-care a step further until you start to feel really replenished. That we'll help you feel more relaxed and energized in the little moments you have, without feeling guilt. We will be better partners,

and mothers, if we focus a little attention on us in the precious minutes we have to ourselves.

Here are some ways my Mom Squad and I kick the self-care
game up a notch:

MAKING SOME ME-TIME

Daphne creates her Me-time in the minutes she has before bed. "I
spend fifteen minutes before bed, every night, doing something that
I love. I was really depressed that I had not pleasure-read for what
felt like years, so I cracked open a new book. It's letting me feed a
love that I used to have that fell by the wayside because kids make
[life] really busy and hectic."

TAKING A BATH

Dr. Morrone: "I take a bath every single night, with candles, because
that's my downtime. And my kids learned, 'It's Mommy's ten-minute
bath time!' I get in the tub, I put my bath salts in, candles, music . . .
I download, and then I'm good to go."

Amber expands on the bathing theme: "If you take a nice bath,
where you soaked in all these oils and salts, and then you go on
Twitter? You're basically reversing the work you just did. Don't
[get] on your phone!"

BUYING YOURSELF SOMETHING NICE

Sometimes self-care involves giving yourself a lovely gift. Amber's
example: "I bought myself this robe after I gave birth to Marlow,
which sounds crazy, but I just wanted to feel a giant warm wrap
around me. I still wear it all the time."

DOING AFFIRMATIONS

Sometimes self-care is about taking care of your mind. Nasiba uses affirmations. "[They're] calming to your brain. My affirmations are more dreamer-type things, like 'I'm going to do this . . . or achieve this . . . or my children are going to be that . . .' It's more like stating and visualizing your dreams." Nasiba also has affirmation cards that she keeps in her bathroom that say things like: "I am doing an amazing job," "I am growth," "I allow my highest good."

Dr. Morrone also feeds the positivity. "I actually subscribe to the DailyOM, and I read it every single day. [Sometimes] I see a good thing to send to my kids, and they're like, 'Okay, would you get us off the mailing list? We're not interested!' And that's where I struggle, because I think, 'This is such a perfect message! How could you not want to read it?'"

A friend of mine uses an app that sends her quotes by poets and philosophers—five times a day—that remind her that she's going to die. The app is inspired by the Bhutanese folk saying, "To be a happy person, one must contemplate death five times a day," and my friend swears by it. So, use whatever kind of affirmation floats your boat! There's a lot out there to choose from.

STAYING FIT

Something else I consider self-care is working out and being active. I used to exercise upon waking, but now that's breakfast time with the kiddo, so as long as I get it done on the early side, I'm good. I have a cycling bike in our bedroom. I lower the lights and do a private SoulCycle class, blasting the music in my headphones and working up a sweat. I prefer exercising in the morning, because I really wake up as soon as I begin to perspire, which takes about fifteen or twenty minutes. Breaking a sweat really sustains me; it helps me shake off the sleep fog—which has gotten more intense with motherhood—and it puts me in a better mood, with more energy. Make a mental note after a workout of your energy and attitude. I'll bet they're both improved!

When I can, I get out to the gym; I like the ritual of it. It reminds me of pre-motherhood days. And while I wouldn't change my current life for the world, it's fun to get back to the gym and work out like I used to.

Beyond working out, the word "fitness" has really taken on a different meaning for me now. I thought I knew what "fitness" was, and, to a certain extent, I did. But it took becoming a mother, being responsible for another person (and not just my partner), to realize that I want to be healthy. Deeply healthy. Not just fit-into-my-dream-jean-size healthy. I want to experience real wellness, over the long haul. My husband and I would like more children, and I plan to be around for their graduations, for their weddings, and to help them raise *their* kids. Do I have the strength, longevity, and stamina for that?

I mentioned earlier that my mother has Alzheimer's disease, and lately, it's not just her mind that's failing her. She has a hard time walking, doctor visits are a regular thing, and she recently had to have another skin cancer spot removed. Her health is something that we, as her children, worry about a lot. I get nervous every time one of my sisters calls me, immediately assuming that it's about my mother.

Soon after I had given birth, I brought Ella to visit my mother; they had met a few times already. When I called to say hello shortly after our visit, my mother told me that my sister-in-law had just had a baby, with obvious grandmotherly pride. But my sister-in-law doesn't have any children; Marjorie was referring to Ella.

I went along with the story, not wanting to confuse her, but this is something that I pray my own children never have to deal with. I want to remain vibrant and fit. Both my partner and I want to be physically and mentally available as long as possible. So fitness, for me, has become less about achieving some perfect ideal and more about building sustainable strength.

When I talked to Mila about this deeper fitness—not just getting back a camera-ready body—her viewpoint had shifted, too. "Yes, my body has changed, but so has my relationship to it. My body has changed, and it'll never be the same. I don't want it to be. I produced two humans out of this body."

With her busy schedule, she also uses her exercising time to be with her husband. "I wake up at 5:30 A.M., I go downstairs with my husband, and we work out together. It's our bonding time. We have the ability to work out at home, [but do] whatever that workout is for you. Get a DVD, get a chair, it doesn't matter. There's no trick to it."

Fit exercise in when you can. I remember one woman on social media telling me she just runs around her backyard in circles during her kids' nap time! However you can fit physical activity into your schedule, do it.

Dee incorporated exercise into time with her kids. "When they went to the park, I played with them. I wasn't the mother who sat on the side; I'd be climbing up on the monkey bars, running around playing tag, so that kept me fit. And you're wearing them out so that when everybody gets home, they're tired."

DAYDREAMING

Speaking of getting tired, every mother I know loves nap time, especially her own. So on days when you can, rest. But resting doesn't always have to be sleeping; another big part of self-care is simple relaxation.

It may sound funny, but one of my favorite things to do is to sit back and daydream. I think of writing ideas, recipes I want to try, places I want to bring my family . . . It's very relaxing and nourishing.

I classify it as self-care because, as mothers, it's not often that we get a moment to just sit and let our minds wander.

DOING WHAT YOU LOVE

I really don't like taking Ella to swim class. I dread schlepping us halfway across town, changing into my bathing suit, and plunking myself into a humid, urine-filled indoor pool. Then I have to do all the drills with her as I get splashed in the face with all the other sweaty moms.

It's just . . . not my thing.

Obviously, there are tasks we do for our kids that don't make us giddy with joy. Zillions of them, in fact. But it's a type of self-care to sit down and have a good think about which activities, in your kid's world, actually make you happy and to try to lean into those. For instance, I love reading books with Ella, showing her stuff in the kitchen makes my heart sing, and I will always volunteer for her daily stroll in the park. Those activities positively light me up inside, and when I'm lit up, I'm a happier person and a better mom.

Jenji Kohan thinks our kids can feel that. "Kids know when you are phoning it in. Know your strong suits. [Don't force] yourself to do things with your kids that you think you *should*, because they know everything. They'll know if you're not enjoying it, and it will affect their fun."

Angela Robinson has a slightly different take on choosing which activities work for her as a parent: "We are kind of unique as a gay family. My wife, Alex, and I embody both mother and father at the same time. Whenever I think of myself as a mother, I think of myself as a mother . . . *plus*."

She laughs.

"Because I'm a little bit Dad. There are all [these] gender

constructs, but Alex will teach him to ski and make sure he's on the swim team, but I cook for the family. It's all a big blender!"

Of course, we can't curate our children's lives to make *us* happy all the time, and, yes, there will be tuba recitals and chess tournaments to attend, but don't be afraid to be honest with yourself about what you enjoy doing and go with it. That's self-care, too.

BEAUTY HACKS

I love a good beauty hack. Here are some of my quick tricks for feeling pretty on a busy schedule.

HAIR

Although my hair is done professionally at work, its natural state is thick, unruly, and, on a humid day, frizzy. My sisters and I affectionately refer to my head of hair as "The Wolf." I was born a redhead, and our hair can be thick, and since I gave birth, it's also become a little coarse, so it can get pretty wild at times.

So I've developed a quick way of taming The Wolf. But no matter the nature of *your* hair, I trust you can adhere to my beauty ethos when it comes to hair hacks: Make the front look good so you can hide the back!

EQUIPMENT

- Spray bottle

- Blow dryer

- Ceramic flat iron hair straightener

- Round brush

- Styling crème (I like Kiehl's Silk Groom. A little goes a long way, and it gives a good "lived in" look.)

Step 1: I dampen the hair all around my hairline by spritzing it with water from the spray bottle. This is the hair in front, around my face, and what I want everyone to focus on.

Step 2: Using the round brush, I get a good grip on a section of damp hair and pull out and down with one hand, following the brush with the dryer in the other hand. This is what we've all seen professional hairdressers do, basically drying and straightening hair at the same time. I continue with all the areas of hair around or near my face, on both sides.

Step 3: Once the hair is dry, I apply the flat iron to all of the sections I've dried, straightening them even more.

Step 4: I part my hair the way I want it, and I squeeze out a tiny, dime-sized amount of styling crème into my palm and rub my hands together. I then run the styling crème lightly over all my hair. It's important to go easy with it; when I use too much, it flattens the whole look and can become greasy, but just enough prevents frizz and gives a nice sheen.

Step 5: Finally, I pull all my hair into a loose, low ponytail or low bun, pulling out some soft tendrils on each side. Because the front of my hair has been tamed, those tendrils look fantastic, and no one even knows the Wolf exists.

COLD WATER FACIAL

This is a trick I've adopted from Mila. She uses it to look refreshed in the morning, and it works wonders when you don't have time for a shower. Just splash icy cold water on your face a few times and then gently pat dry. It helps the puffiness go down and jolts me awake. Good morning!

If you do have time for a shower and are feeling especially bold, turn the faucet to cold for your final rinse. It might make you shriek a little, but it's guaranteed to wake you up, and the cold water tightens your pores.

THE MINI-MAKEOVER

As mothers, we just don't have the primping time we used to. Here are my super-quick tips for looking lovely (or at least not so exhausted) without putting in the hours. It's a six-step process that should take less than five minutes. I like this routine for when I'm just running around doing errands but I want to look awake and a teeny bit glam. Try it!

Step 1: I apply a little concealer around my eyes, especially if I haven't slept enough.

Step 2: I give my eyebrows some love. Mine are naturally light in color, so that means filling them in and shaping with an eyebrow brush.

Step 3: I apply a little contour under my cheekbones for definition—with a little on my cheeks for bronzing—and use the same contour on my eyelid crease.

Step 4: I curl my eyelashes. This is a game changer. Curling my lashes opens up my eyes, making me look more awake and refreshed. My favorite curler is by Shu Uemura, and it's the best I've ever used. Just order one on Amazon. It will become another good friend.

Step 5: I use one coat of mascara.

Step 6: I apply lip gloss.

DONE.

Combined with the hair hack (above), this mini-makeover takes me through the whole day feeling like a presentable human being!

TOOLS FOR SELF-CARE

- Making some Me-time

- Taking a bath

- Buying yourself something nice

- Doing affirmations

- Staying fit

- Daydreaming

- Doing what you love

- Beauty hacks

If you've struggled with self-care, you're not alone. But you are central to the lives of everyone in your family, and when you receive some TLC, everyone benefits.

So start drawing that bath!

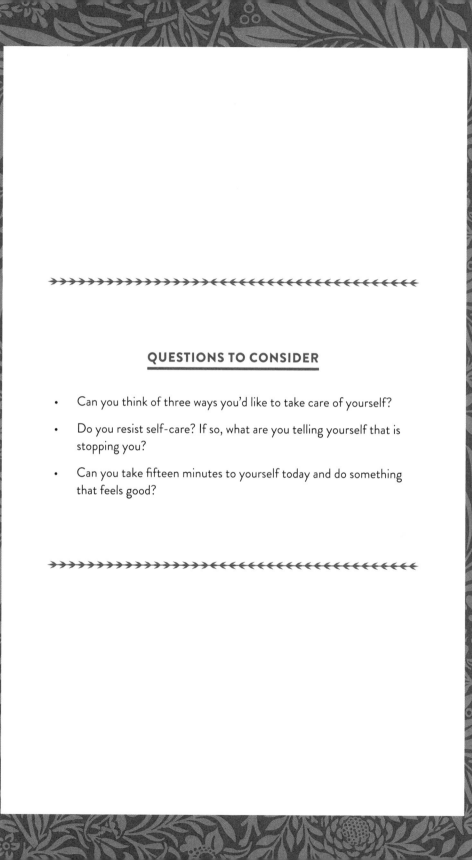

QUESTIONS TO CONSIDER

- Can you think of three ways you'd like to take care of yourself?

- Do you resist self-care? If so, what are you telling yourself that is stopping you?

- Can you take fifteen minutes to yourself today and do something that feels good?

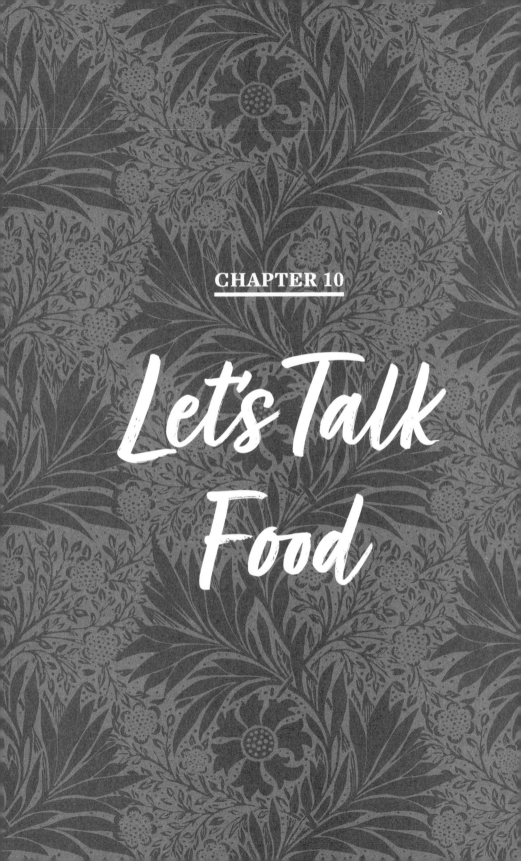

CHAPTER 10

Let's Talk
Food

THE NOURISHMENT NITTY-GRITTY

Food is a really big part of my life. Thanks to my mom, Marjorie, I was introduced to some delicious, exotic cuisines as a kid, and I have always loved cooking, being in the kitchen, and sharing meals with others.

But a number of years ago I began experiencing some mysterious health symptoms, including joint pain, digestive issues, and extremely low energy. I found myself going from expert to expert, trying to get a handle on them. I went from Western medical doctors to "woo-woo" practitioners, from specialists for specific ailments to doctors who weren't in the phone book or on Yelp. I floated in sensory deprivation tanks (or saltwater tanks), ate alkaline for months on end, endured thermographic body scans, did metaphysical work, and had my blood projected from a microscope onto a very large screen in order to detect parasites.

You name it, I did it.

A nd the one common denominator I discovered, among all these modalities, was this: What we put in our bodies *matters*. More specifically, food matters. Food has the power to keep us vibrant, energized, and happy. And the more whole a food is, the more power it has.

From then on I brought this wisdom into my life. I focused my passion for cooking on cleaner, healthier fare. I started playing with whole grains and more vegetables, sourcing food at the local farmers markets, and drinking bone broths. I really began to listen to what my body was telling me.

And I got better. The pain and digestive issues improved drastically. I had more energy and lost stubborn weight. I wrote about all this in *The Stash Plan*, so I won't go into great detail here, but suffice it to say that by immersing myself in healthy eating and learning how the body works (my first book also focused on the liver and gall bladder), I really turned my life around. It was a long journey but one that was satisfying, enlightening, and absolutely worthwhile.

Since I gave birth to Ella, my food habits have had to change radically. I now revolve my life, and my eating, around a little redhead's schedule, and that's a big shift. And that's on *top* of working around my husband's timetable, tending to my own work life, squeezing in fitness, making room for our partnership, and enjoying some shred of a social life.

I've had to adapt. I've had to learn how to nourish myself and my family using methods that are quick, easy, and flexible. And, sure, I want to look good and maintain a slim figure, but this is about more than that. As I mentioned in the previous chapter about going deeper with my fitness, I want to go deeper with nutrition, too. I want a type of nourishment that produces profound wellness and will keep us around for a long time.

Becoming a mom made me rethink my priorities and get realistic about what I *must* do and what I can let slide. Based on my years of trial and error, plus the wisdom I've garnered from experts, I've boiled nourishment down to a couple of personal bottom lines. By adhering to these, I can keep us

Food has the power to keep us vibrant, energized, and happy.

fueled for the wonderful chaos of family life, knowing that I'm also protecting our bodies. No matter how depleted or tired or pulled in different directions I am, I do my best to maintain these standards.

My bottom lines are:

- Eating organic foods whenever possible

- Drinking bone broth regularly

BOTTOM LINE #1: EATING ORGANIC FOOD

I talk a lot about the importance of eating organically: on social media, on my YouTube channel, in interviews, to my husband and child, with friends and siblings—basically to anybody within close proximity!

I feel it's *that* important. Here's why:

By eating organic foods, I avoid two things: genetically modified organisms (GMOs) and—perhaps more critically—the chemicals sprayed on them.

Here's a little history:

When GMO soy and corn were introduced into the American food supply in 1996, they were genetically designed to withstand a particular weed killer called glyphosate. This breakthrough allowed farmers, who had previously been careful with the stuff, to spray tons and tons of glyphosate on their fields without killing their crops.

And I mean *tons.*

Since then, the worldwide use of glyphosate has multiplied a mind-blowing fifteen times.[1] Within the United States, we've gone from applying less than twenty-five million pounds of glyphosate on our crops in 1992 to nearly three hundred million pounds in 2016.[2]

That's a twelvefold increase in *fourteen* years.

And it's no longer just corn and soy that have been genetically modified. Since the turn of the century, we've also introduced glyphosate-resistant GMO canola, cotton, sorghum, sugar beets,

GMOS PLAY HIDE-AND-SEEK

Ella's new obsession is crackers. Recently she picked up a package of a very popular brand-name cracker in the store, and I looked at its list of ingredients. Among the top eight were soybean oil, sugar, partially hydrogenated cottonseed oil, high fructose corn syrup, and soy lecithin. Considering that more than 90 percent of the corn, soy, and cotton grown in America is genetically modified to be glyphosate resistant,[3] and about half of all sugar we use comes from genetically modified sugar beets,[4] those crackers definitely would have exposed her to glyphosate!

It can be tricky navigating the marketplace, as so many items and ingredients are derived from these crops. Here's a handy list of ingredients that are derived from corn:

- Citric acid
- Confectioners' sugar
- Corn flour
- Corn fructose
- Cornmeal
- Corn oil
- Corn syrup
- Dextrin and dextrose
- Fructose
- High fructose corn syrup
- Lactic acid
- Malt
- Mono- and diglycerides
- Monosodium glutamate
- Sorbitol
- Starch

and alfalfa to the market and our tables. And considering that derivatives of many of these foods are found in practically every processed food (see sidebar), the average American family is being exposed to lots and lots of glyphosate without their knowledge or permission. When tested for, glyphosate has shown up in rainwater, groundwater, the air, food products, the Great Barrier Reef, and even human urine.[5]

But what's glyphosate doing to us?

In 2001, microbiologist Joshua Lederberg brought the term "microbiome" into the mainstream when he described the teeming, thriving world of microorganisms that lives in our guts. Little did

And these items/ingredients are made (or can be made) from soy:

Bulking agents

Emulsifiers

Guar gum

Natural flavors

Shoyu

Soy beverages

Soy flour

Soy lecithin

Soy miso

Soy protein concentrate or isolate

Soy sauce

Soybean oil

Stabilizer

Tamari

- Tempeh
- Tofu
- Texturized vegetable protein
- Vegetable broth
- Vegetable gum

And like I mentioned above, whenever you see "sugar" on a label, there's a fifty-fifty chance it comes from a glyphosate-resistant GMO beet.

You don't eat alfalfa? That's cool, but the cow whose meat you and your family ate probably munched on it (and if not, she certainly ate feed made from GMO soy and/or corn). Chickens are also routinely fed soy, corn, or their derivatives.

And those potato chips you're noshing on? There's a good chance they were fried in GMO cottonseed oil.

Sorry. Ugh.

we know that we play host to *ten times* as many bacterial cells as we do human ones in our intestines alone. And it turns out these bacteria play a critical role in our digestion, immune system response, and even our mental health. To put it simply, when our gut critters are out of balance, *we* are out of balance.

Although it's considered unethical to make humans ingest a pesticide for the purposes of science, researchers have been looking at what glyphosate does to animals and their microbiomes. A study conducted at the University of Texas at Austin found that glyphosate destroyed specialized gut bacteria in bees, leaving them more susceptible to infection and death and possibly playing a role in colony collapse.[6] When studying the microorganisms in the guts of chickens, scientists found that good bacteria were destroyed by glyphosate, while dangerous bacteria were resistant to it.[7] In fish, exposure to glyphosate brought about the symptoms of celiac disease,[8] and researchers in Italy found that when prepubescent rats were given glyphosate in doses considered safe, the experiment "resulted in significant and distinctive changes in overall bacterial composition."[9]

Could those changes be happening to us, too?

Well, when we look at the twenty-plus years that we've been going crazy with glyphosate, the incidence of certain conditions has increased at an alarming speed. Crohn's disease and celiac disease have been on a steady rise, while rates of food allergies, ADHD, obesity, and many autoimmune diseases—all of which are connected to gut health—have exploded as well.[10]

And there seems to be a growing connection between glyphosate and cancer. In March 2015 the World Health Organization's International Agency for Research on Cancer unanimously determined that glyphosate is "probably carcinogenic to humans," and in 2019 a man suffering from non-Hodgkin's lymphoma—who'd used glyphosate at his job—was awarded $289 million in damages by a San Francisco jury (later reduced to $78 million on appeal).[11] In the same year, a couple who had both been diagnosed with non-Hodgkin's lymphoma were awarded a stunning $2 *billion* after they'd made the case that their conditions were caused by the world's most popular (glyphosate-based) herbicide.

Whether these are simply scary coincidences or not, I don't want my family participating in this informal study.

So, yeah, that's why I stick with organic foods. If you're interested in knowing more on this topic, I cover it extensively in *The Stash Plan*. I stress the importance of organic eating because the federal standards put out by the USDA certify that when a food is labeled "USDA Organic," it contains neither GMOs nor glyphosate. I feel that, as a mother, it's the safest choice I can make for my family.

Whenever I post from the farmers market on social media, inevitably a few people will remark on how expensive the organic food I buy there must be. And it *can* be more expensive, although that isn't always the case these days. For instance, do you know that the biggest seller of organic food in this country is Costco?[12]

That's right. *Costco.*

Eating organically has become so popular in the

LABEL WATCHING

You may also see foods with a "No GMOs" sticker or a logo that states Non-GMO Project. Because U.S. companies are not (yet) required to reveal their GMO usage, at least the ones that *refrain* from using GMOs can show off their status. But remember: Just because a food isn't genetically modified doesn't mean it wasn't sprayed with chemicals. In fact, one of the most common uses of glyphosate is as a desiccant that dries out crops so that they're ready for harvest. It is regularly used on (non-GMO) wheat and oats. Considering that oatmeal and whole wheat bread are staples in my home, I'm so grateful to know this.

last couple of decades that the market is finally bringing the prices down, and Costco is a part of that. And obviously the competition has to keep up, so, having purchased Whole Foods Market, Amazon has also lowered the price on produce of all kinds. Trader Joe's has many organic products, and even Walmart is in the game, with a wide selection of organics. When it comes to processed foods, like snacks, crackers, noodles, etc., there seems to be an organic version of just about everything these days.

I recently sat down with Jeffrey Smith, a consumer activist and author of two books and two documentaries on the dangers of genetically modified foods. He's a big proponent of organic foods, and I asked him many questions. The first was:

Can everyone afford organic food?

"First of all, if someone is buying processed foods, and they switch from conventional processed to organic processed, that's the [most expensive] category. If they're buying ingredients and *making* food, then it's much easier and it's less expensive."

Jeffrey also offers another great way of looking at the economics of organic food:

"Here's what I suggest to people. Combine three budgets: your health budget, your food budget, and your philanthropy budget."

***Philanthropy* budget?**

"When we spend money on organic food, we are reducing the number of pesticides in the ground and increasing biodiversity. It builds the entire ecosystem—insects, the microbial [world], the downstream effects, even the weather is affected—so if you think in terms of how much you could spend as a *donor* each year, you can stick some of that into your organic food spending."

So buying organic food is like making a daily donation to the environment, because the choices we make have ripple effects. When I buy from local organic farmers, I am supporting individuals who work their butts off protecting the soil, the water, and the planet. They're simply doing the right thing.

What about the health budget?

"I interviewed a family for the film *Secret Ingredients*. Six people in the family, with an eighteen-thousand-dollar-per-year medical bill. After a year of organic [eating], it was nine thousand dollars. After two years, it was three thousand. Just their premiums! The kids no longer go to the doctors' except for annual checkups. The savings in terms of money spent on medical [expenses] is often substantial. And it's real."

I asked Jeffrey about the different ways consumers could integrate organic foods and products into their lives:

"There are some people who hear this information, and they get immediately to the 'cupboard stage,' where they go and throw things out. There are other people who say, 'Okay, I'm not throwing anything out, but everything new that I buy [will be organic].' Then there are some who are more selective: 'I can't afford *all* organic, so I need to come up with a list of what the most important things are.' And so, everyone's going to be different. The recommendation is to try to go one hundred percent organic, if you can, for a month, and see what happens to your life!"

And what has he seen when people do that?

"It is predictable: The number one improvement is always in digestive disorders. Number two is increased energy and brain function. Eighty-two to eighty-five percent showed improvements in digestion, and over sixty percent in fatigue and weight. Weight loss is huge."

Understanding the dangers of GMOs and glyphosate, as well as the value of organic food, I feel empowered to make really good choices for myself and my family, choices that will protect our health—physically, mentally, and emotionally—for the rest of

THE MOMMY DOLLAR

You and I as moms have a lot of power. According to *Forbes*, 85 percent of all household purchases are made by mothers, and altogether we spend 2.4 *trillion* dollars annually.[13] Considering that the entire American economy—including all personal, corporate, and government spending—is just over $20 trillion, ours is a significant slice of the pie. What you and I choose to buy—and, just as important, *not* to buy—can shift an entire market.

Led by Jeffrey Smith, the Institute for Responsible Technology has been reaching out to educate moms about GMOs and organics for quite a while:

"They've been our number one priority for years, and that has caused the tipping point in the United States. Forty-six percent of Americans say they're trying to avoid GMOs, and now major food companies are scrambling to replace brands more and more with non-GMO ingredients."

See? We're powerful!

And Jeffrey understands how our Version 2.0 brains work:

"It came from framing the debate about the health dangers, so it wasn't a boycott; it was realizing that using the [nonorganic] foods could damage their child. Moms are pre-wired to protect their kids, so they can make excuses for themselves, [but] it's harder to make excuses for their kids."

So just know that every time you spend a dollar, it counts. It's noticed. And it's shifting the economy. And when we pool all our dollars, making the purchases that support our children—while also causing awesome ripple effects in the environment—we are building a healthier, cleaner, better place to live.

That's a Mommy Dollar world.

our lives. *That's* why buying organic food is a bottom line I do my utmost not to cross.

BOTTOM LINE #2: DRINKING BONE BROTH

My second bottom line—and another common denominator among most of the wellness experts I've seen—is drinking lots of bone broth. In my experience, among those who work with the body, bone broth is acknowledged and respected for its health benefits.

The first time I had a cup of homemade bone broth, I felt as if my cells perked up and thanked me. It felt primal, like my DNA craved it. It wasn't until I started drinking bone broth that I felt deeply nourished, my body got stronger, and my digestion improved. At the same time, I started to look better and feel better, and my skin became all glowy and vibrant.

Bone broths have been around for millennia. The original broths were actually stone soups, made to leach the minerals from rocks, but as humans became better hunters, bones and other foods were added. Eventually, bone broth was associated with healing. Many different types of broths are used in Chinese medicine, and the great Jewish scholar Maimonides recommended chicken soup to treat the sick way back in twelfth-century Egypt. Today, broths are daily fare throughout Asia, while much of French cuisine is based on excellent bouillons and broths, and "cow foot soup" is considered a medicinal drink in parts of the Caribbean.[14] Whether it's called *cocido* (Mexico) or *kholodets* (Russia), bone broth shows up just about everywhere.

WHAT IS BONE BROTH?

Just like it sounds, bone broth is a soup made from extracting the minerals, vitamins, marrow, and collagen from animal bones. Together, these create a powerful elixir. You can use beef, chicken, fish (or any other kind of animal) bones, simmered with lots of vegetables and herbs, for up to twenty-four hours (recipe coming up). The bones should be from grass-fed, organic livestock raised without antibiotics. If you're vegan or vegetarian, a hearty vegetable broth—that includes some seaweed—can also deliver a healing, micronutrient punch.

By letting a broth simmer for hours, all the goodness from the bones and vegetables is integrated into the liquid and then can go straight to your intestines, to be absorbed easily and quickly into the bloodstream. There's no chewing or gas or effort involved.

You can find some really good bone broths at better health food stores.* so you don't always have to make your own. But try it at least once. It's so easy! There is nothing more grounding than firing up some bone broth and letting it do its thing in my slow cooker. I feel like I'm connecting with my ancestors.

Let's take a look at the benefits of bone broth:

Bone broth supports the gut: Because it contains an amino acid called glutamine, bone broth helps heal the tiny hairlike protrusions (called villi) along the walls of the intestine that absorb nutrients.

And since the intestine is made of its own kind of internal "skin," the collagen in bone broth supports both the gut lining and its overall elasticity, strengthening it while inhibiting permeability. Speaking of collagen . . .

Bone broth delivers collagen: The most abundant type of protein in our bodies, collagen keeps our skin plump and beautiful.

---

* I'm talking about recently cooked broth, made by local companies. If it's in a box or a can, take a pass.

But as we age, we naturally lose collagen, and most women I know (myself included) have used creams and lotions containing some sort of collagen in order to keep our youthful-looking skin. But bone broth does just that, from the inside out!

And that's not all: Collagen sort of holds everything together like glue. In addition to skin, collagen is found in our bones, muscles, and tendons, and it's what gives us flexibility, keeping our bodies supple. If you maintain your collagen through regular bone-broth drinking, your joints will stay lubricated, and your bones will be stronger.

Bone broth supports the immune system (in a few ways): First, bone broth reduces inflammation in the gut, which gives your immune system a much-needed rest. Second, bone broth contains an amino acid called arginine, which is critical to liver function and immunity from disease. Finally, because bones house bone marrow—which contains fats called alkylglycerols—bone broth supports the production of white blood cells, vital to our immune system response. FYI: Alkylglycerols are also found in colostrum and have been found to suppress tumor growth. Go, alkylglycerols!

When I first started incorporating bone broth into my diet, my health was pretty compromised, so I had three cups a day—one with each meal. I would drink it like a tea. These days I have one cup a day, usually with lunch. When I'm working, I bring it along in a travel mug.

My family has bone broth daily as well. Most of our proteins and grains are cooked in it, and I always have broth or a big soup in our fridge. As soon as I got the okay from our pediatrician, I was giving Ella bone broth in a bottle, and now her favorite foods are the soups I make for her from broth. Even when I make her a sandwich, she always wants a bowl of broth or soup to dip it in.

THE 80:20 RULE

I have my bottom lines, but that doesn't mean I follow them perfectly all the time. There will be food in restaurants that isn't organic; Ella will get stuff at school or birthday parties that I can't control. And later, when she's in high school . . . well, we'll cross that bridge when we come to it.

Life is life, and we spent a whole chapter discussing how we need to practice letting go sometimes. I'm not here to wag a finger but to offer information, so you can make your own decisions about your own bottom lines.

And follow them imperfectly.

I try to live by the 80:20 rule: If I follow my principles 80 percent of the time, I give myself permission to ease up the other 20. Life is always changing, and I need to keep some flexibility in the system. Without that, I set myself up for inner conflict and stressing out the people around me.

I like to have a Cheat Night every once in a while, and I usually save it for an evening my husband and I have together. We can go to a new restaurant, try some fancy foods, and I get to relax my rules a bit. I know that by living by my bottom lines *most* of the time—and always in my own household—I'm building the life I want to live. The rest of the time? I relax and enjoy.

>>>>>>>>>>>>>>>>>>>>>>>>>>>>><<<<<<<<<<<<<<<<<<<<<<<<<<<<<

QUESTIONS TO CONSIDER

- What changed in your food life when you became a mom?

- Do you have your own personal nourishment bottom lines? If not, are you willing to consider some?

- Are there cost-effective ways you can introduce more organic food into the family fare?

- Are you curious about bone broth?

>>>>>>>>>>>>>>>>>>>>>>>>>>>>><<<<<<<<<<<<<<<<<<<<<<<<<<<<<

CHAPTER 11

Recipes

Just as the sun rises every morning, so do families. Stomachs grumble, and households crank up into action; food needs to get into mouths, *stat.*

Here are some delicious recipes that will help you nourish your family. The first section includes meals that get the whole family together. The second section covers some tried-and-true basics that I keep going back to, especially since becoming a mother. In the third section are recipes for children's ever-evolving palates, and, finally, some recipes for those special evenings with your partner.

I've also created labels that may show up on some of the recipes. They are as follows:

- Batch Cook: These recipes are great for bigger batches.

- Freezer Friendly: These recipes can be frozen and reheated later.

- Trojan Foods: These recipes offer opportunities to sneak healthy ingredients, like vegetables, into unsuspecting children. Mwahaha.

As I've just mentioned in the previous chapter, I recommend you use organic ingredients whenever possible, including for your oils, herbs, and spices.

And finally, because I cook for a toddler, I tend to go very light on the seasoning at first and then add more later, for the adults. If any of my recipes are too lightly seasoned for you or your family, adjust to suit your tastes and needs.

Bon appétit!

FAMILY DINNERS

Main Course Salad

Serves 4

Many of the crew on the set of *Orange*—the people responsible for moving all of the trucks and trailers and picking up actors and so on—were members of the Teamsters Union. Most of them were men with amazingly thick New York accents who made me feel right at home. After *The Stash Plan* came out, a few of the Teamsters started telling me what they were eating, almost like they were at confession. "Laura, I only had *one* donut today with my cawfee," said one. I would laugh and say, "That's good!" A couple of weeks later, the same brawny guy told me that instead of having a donut, he'd had oatmeal for breakfast. "That's great!" I chirped. A week later: "Laura, I had a salad for lunch . . . I got it with the Quoon-wee!" he said. There was a pause. "You mean *quinoa*?" I asked. "Yeah!" he exclaimed, and I laughed at his excitement. "We got the quinoa and all the surroundin's," he said, by which he meant all the fixings around the lettuce. I loved that. And ever since then, I refer to the salad fixings as "surroundin's."

This is the greens mixture I usually do, but you can include any greens you like.

➤➤➤➤➤➤➤➤➤➤➤➤➤➤➤➤➤➤➤➤➤◄◄◄◄◄◄◄◄◄◄◄◄◄◄◄◄◄◄◄◄◄

SALAD

6 cups mixed greens

1 cup spinach leaves

1 cup frisée (optional—this lettuce can be bitter)

1 cup chopped iceberg lettuce

SURROUNDIN'S

2 cups cooked brown rice, quinoa, or other grain

Chopped tomatoes

Shredded cheese

Toasted pine nuts

Sliced cucumber

Sliced radishes

Some kind of protein, such as cooked sliced chicken breast, ground turkey, or sliced steak

Cooked and crumbled bacon

DRESSING

1 small clove garlic (if you have a large clove, use half a clove)

½ teaspoon plus a pinch of salt

Juice of ½ lemon

½ cup extra virgin olive oil

¼ teaspoon ground black pepper

½ teaspoon Dijon mustard

½ teaspoon maple syrup

>>>>>>>>>>>>>>>>>>>><<<<<<<<<<<<<<<<<<<<<<<

TO MAKE THE SALAD

In a salad bowl, toss the greens. Set aside.

TO MAKE THE DRESSING

Using a mortar and pestle (or a Japanese suribachi—a ridged mortar with wooden pestle), muddle the garlic with a pinch of salt until the garlic turns into a thin paste. Add the lemon juice and mix to incorporate all the garlic from the mortar. Transfer to a bowl, add the remaining ½ teaspoon salt and the pepper, then slowly whisk in the oil until emulsified. Whisk in the mustard and maple syrup. Taste and adjust the seasonings according to your preference.

Fill everyone's bowls with the salad and lay all the surroundin's in bowls with serving spoons down the middle of the table. Let everyone mix and match to their preference.

Dig in and enjoy!

VARIATION

For a spicy, creamier version of the dressing, whisk in ¼ teaspoon wasabi powder and 2 teaspoons mayonnaise. If you love a good kick, add even more wasabi!

Taco Night

Makes 12 tacos • Taco meat: Batch Cook

This recipe is inspired by Jenji. She likes to do interactive dinners that bring her family together, and Taco Night is one of their household faves. With tacos you can pick and choose exactly what you want. And they make a great spread if your kids have different tastes and needs, which was the case in Jenji's house. "My boys had really severe allergies, and my daughter would only want to eat things that would kill them," she says, so she developed a way that everyone could choose what they wanted, staying happy and healthy!

TACO FILLING

1 tablespoon salted butter

1 tablespoon olive oil

¼ red bell pepper, seeded and peeled, finely chopped

1 clove garlic, finely chopped

1 small shallot, finely chopped

1 pound ground chicken, beef, or turkey

1 packet organic taco seasoning

2 tablespoons plain tomato sauce (don't use marinara, because it's seasoned)

¼ to ½ cup bone broth (if I'm making beef tacos, I use beef broth; for chicken or turkey tacos, I use chicken broth)

2 teaspoons ground cumin

1 teaspoon sea salt

SURROUNDIN'S

12 taco shells (1 box) or soft tortillas

Sliced avocado or guacamole

Seeded and chopped tomatoes

Chopped fresh cilantro

Salsa

Sour cream

Sliced (into thin strips) iceberg lettuce

2 cups grated cheddar cheese

Hot sauce (optional)

Preheat the oven to 350°F.

TO MAKE THE TACO FILLING

Melt the butter in the oil in a large skillet over medium-low heat. Add the bell pepper, garlic, and shallot and cook for about 5 minutes, stirring often, until the shallot is softened and translucent. Add the meat, taco seasoning, tomato sauce, ¼ cup bone broth, the cumin, and salt and increase the heat to medium. Chop with the flat end of a wooden spoon or spatula to break up the meat and mix in the taco seasoning. Bring to a simmer and cook for 5 to 7 minutes, until the meat is cooked through, adding more broth if the meat starts to dry out (I sometimes find this happens with chicken and turkey). Remove from the heat and set aside.

TO MAKE THE SURROUNDIN'S

If you're using taco shells, place them on a baking sheet, place in the oven, and warm for 5 minutes. Here's a tip: I layer the shells loosely inside one another and gently wedge a metal ¼-cup or ½-cup measuring cup into the last shell to keep it open so they don't close up like a clamshell! (Be careful when you remove them from the oven, as the metal measuring cup gets very hot.)

If you're using soft tortillas, wrap them in stacks of six in parchment-lined tinfoil, place in the oven, and warm for 10 minutes. Remove from the oven and wrap them in a slightly dampened clean dishtowel to keep them warm and soft.

Place the filling and all the surroundin's in pretty dishes in the middle of the table with serving spoons. Dig in!

VARIATIONS

- You can use all these ingredients the next day for a great taco salad.
- I've also heated broth with the taco meat, added chopped spinach and rice, and thrown it into a thermos for an awesome nutritious soup on the go.

Pho

Serves 4

This recipe is inspired by Nasiba, who, like me, always has a stash of bone broth in the fridge or freezer. It's the main component of this delicious, traditional Vietnamese dish. Part of the fun of this meal is putting it together, so assign family members different tasks to make the surroundin's.

SOUP

8 cups Chicken Broth (page 181) or Beef Broth (page 184)

1-inch piece ginger

1½ tablespoons Bragg Liquid Aminos

2 cloves garlic, peeled and chopped

1 tablespoon umeboshi plum vinegar

Pad Thai rice noodles

SURROUNDIN'S (MAKE SOME OR ALL)

1 teaspoon baking soda

Chopped broccoli

Chopped cauliflower

Snow peas

Carrots, peeled and sliced into ½-inch rounds

Mushrooms, sliced,

Thinly sliced cooked chicken, beef, and/or tofu

Perfect Yellow Hard-Boiled Eggs (page 177), sliced

Fresh Thai basil leaves

Bean sprouts

Fresh mint leaves

Chopped fresh cilantro

Lime wedges

Hoisin sauce

Srir acha sauce

Bragg Liquid Aminos or soy sauce

Combine the broth, ginger, liquid aminos, garlic, and vinegar in a large pot and bring to a simmer over medium heat. Simmer for 5 minutes, then reduce the heat to low and cover, letting it continue to cook and have flavors meld together.

While the broth continues to cook, make the noodles according to the package instructions. Strain and transfer the noodles to a bowl filled with fresh water (this prevents them from sticking together and becoming a gluey mess).

Add a few inches of water to a large saucepan. Place a steamer on top (make sure it doesn't touch the water) and bring to a simmer over medium heat. Once the steam starts coming up, add the baking soda to the water (this makes the colors of the vegetables pop!). Steam broccoli, cauliflower, snow peas, and carrots separately in batches for about 2 to 3 minutes or until they reach your desired doneness. Place into separate bowls on the dinner table, along with separate bowls for the mushrooms and proteins. Set out the basil, bean sprouts, mint, cilantro, and lime wedges all together on a plate or in separate bowls, depending on how picky your kids are. Set out the hoisin sauce, sriracha, and liquid aminos.

Place a handful of noodles into each serving bowl and spoon the hot broth over them. Have everyone choose their own toppings. Slurp and enjoy!

THE BASICS

Oatmeal, Three Ways

Serves 4 • Batch Cook

I love using steel-cut oats for my morning oatmeal because they are the closest things to the original oat groats, but they cook much faster. I find them more satisfying than rolled or quick oats because they have a coarser, chewier texture. The more whole a grain is, the more slowly its glucose is absorbed into the bloodstream, which helps you to feel fuller, longer. And you can't beat the lovely nutty taste of a steel-cut oat.

How do I make my oatmeal "quick" while keeping its nutrients, flavor, and texture? I make it ahead of time then slowly reheat it with homemade almond milk (see page 174). It tastes amazing and is a great base for adding whatever you and your family like.

>>>>>>>>>>>>>>>>>>>>><<<<<<<<<<<<<<<<<<<<<<

1 cup steel-cut oats (use gluten-free oats if you are avoiding gluten)

4 cups water

1 teaspoon salted butter

1 teaspoon sea salt (I use Real Salt or Himalayan salt)

>>>>>>>>>>>>>>>>>>>>><<<<<<<<<<<<<<<<<<<<<<

In a medium nonstick saucepan, combine the oats and water and bring to a boil. Reduce the heat to maintain a simmer and cover, leaving a slight space for steam to escape and avoid bubbling over. Cook for about 20 minutes, stirring a few times so it cooks evenly and doesn't stick to the bottom, until oats are cooked through and are the desired texture.

Add the butter and salt, cover again, remove from the heat, and let sit for a few minutes. Stir before serving.

Here are the three ways I like to serve it:

1. For me: I mix in a scoop of collagen powder (I get it from the grocery store or health food store), 2 tablespoons almond milk, and 1 teaspoon peanut butter and top it with chopped walnuts and almonds. Sometimes I will add chocolate protein powder in place of the collagen powder for a chocolaty–peanut butter flavor.

2. For my daughter: I add fresh berries or half a sliced banana and drizzle with a teaspoon of maple syrup. She likes hers sweet.

3. For my husband: I top it with salt and freshly cracked black pepper, sliced avocado, and chopped walnuts. He likes a savory breakfast.

FYI

- I like to cook oatmeal in a nonstick pot because it makes cleanup a lot easier.
- When I batch, I double this recipe.
- To reheat, I put a few scoops of oats into a pot with homemade almond milk (recipe follows) and a touch of honey and heat over medium-low heat. I chop the oats with the flat end of a spatula; as they heat up with the almond milk, they break apart to return to oatmeal consistency.

Almond Milk

Makes 6 cups • Batch Cook

This is so easy to make that I always have some in the fridge. When I transitioned my daughter from breast milk, I often gave her homemade almond milk and she still drinks it every day. I use it for my oats, with other cereals, and in my cold brew in the morning. It requires a nut milk bag, which you can find on Amazon or in kitchen stores.

>>>>>>>>>>>>>>>>>>><<<<<<<<<<<<<<<<<<<<<<<

2 cups raw almonds   Water

>>>>>>>>>>>>>>>>>>><<<<<<<<<<<<<<<<<<<<<<<

Soak the almonds in a bowl with water (covered by an inch) for about 8 hours or overnight. Pour through a strainer, discarding the water, and rinse the almonds. Place the almonds in a blender with 5 cups fresh water and blend well to the consistency of whole milk. Depending on the size of your blender, make in batches. Place a nut milk bag in a large bowl. Pour the mixture into the nut bag and squeeze out your fresh almond milk!

Discard the ground almond pulp, or use it to make almond-pulp crackers, baked goods, or other yummy things. There are lots of recipes online.

Cold-Brew Coffee "Moonshine"

Makes 8 cups

My lifestyle often demands a lot of coffee; it's not unusual for me to be up for work at 4 A.M. and then put in a sixteen- to eighteen-hour day. So coffee is important, and its taste and quality matter. I prefer cold brew, because it's 60 percent less acidic than hot-brewed coffee, making it way easier on my stomach. I think every mom should know about it. Here's the recipe for my morning moonshine.

>>>>>>>>>>>>>>>>>>>>><<<<<<<<<<<<<<<<<<<<<

Equipment I use for this recipe:

Toddy Cold Brew System*	Water
Coffee grinder	Ice cubes
12-ounce bag of your favorite coffee beans	Almond milk or other milk or cream (optional)
	Simple Syrup (recipe follows)

>>>>>>>>>>>>>>>>>>>>><<<<<<<<<<<<<<<<<<<<<

Grind the coffee beans in batches for 7 seconds** and place in a bowl.

Place the stopper and the filter in the bottom of the coffee maker. Pour half of the ground coffee into the Toddy and add 4 cups filtered water. Let sit for 5 minutes. Add the rest of the coffee grinds and another 4 cups filtered water. Gently stir to mix. Let sit overnight.

In the morning, place the Toddy coffee maker holding the coffee over the glass canister (part of the Toddy system) securely. Carefully release the

---

* This Toddy system is what I've found works well. You can find it online for roughly $35. Feel free to try other brands!

** I find that 7 seconds creates the perfect consistency for me—not too fine that it clogs the Toddy filter, and not so coarse that it won't release its goodness. Grinders can vary, so find the perfect amount of grind time for you.

stopper at the bottom, allowing the cold-brewed coffee to filter through into the glass container below. When done, discard the coffee grounds, rinse the filter, and put it in a storage baggie in the refrigerator. It can be reused multiple times. I've experimented many ways to prolong the life of the filter, and the best way I've found is to store it in a little baggie while it's wet in the fridge until next time.

Place ice in your favorite mug or vessel (I like a Mason jar) and pour your desired amount of coffee over it. Remember, this is a concentrated brew, so you will want to add some filtered water to taste. Add almond milk (or other cream/milk) and simple syrup (recipe follows) to taste. Stir well (I put the lid on the jar and shake vigorously to get a foam on top). Yum!

Store the rest of the cold-brew in a sealed glass container in the fridge.

Simple Syrup

Makes about 1½ cups

I love this recipe because it is SO easy! I can't tell you how many friends were blown away that I make my own simple syrup; they thought it was something you can only find in a gourmet coffee shop. When I showed them how easy it is, they all started making it.

1 cup water   1 cup turbinado sugar

In a small saucepan, combine the water and ½ cup of the sugar. Place over medium-high heat and slowly stir constantly until the sugar dissolves. Add the remaining ½ cup of the sugar and stir until it dissolves. Do not let it come to a boil. This will only take a few minutes. Let cool completely, then transfer to a glass jar, cover, and refrigerate.

Perfect Yellow Hard-Boiled Eggs

Makes 12

As a working mother, I need quick protein grabs, ready at any time. Luckily, fresh eggs from a farmers market can last up to a month in the fridge, making hard-boiled eggs an easy protein go-to that can be made ahead of time. However, using the wrong technique can turn the yolk gray and dry. This is a foolproof recipe I've used since I was ten years old. Thanks to my mother, I've never had a gray yolk since . . . as long as I'm cooking it!

>>>>>>>>>>>>>>>>>>>>>><<<<<<<<<<<<<<<<<<<<<<<<<

12 fresh eggs	Salt and ground black pepper

>>>>>>>>>>>>>>>>>>>>>><<<<<<<<<<<<<<<<<<<<<<<<<

Place the eggs in a large pot and add water to cover by 1 to 2 inches. Place over high heat and bring to a rolling boil. The boil is very important. You want the water boiling so strongly that the bubbles are rolling over the top of the water and the eggs are hoppin' and poppin' on the bottom of the pot. When you think the water is at a rolling boil, count to five. At five, cover and immediately remove from the heat.

Set a timer for 15 minutes. After 10 minutes have elapsed, fill a medium bowl with ice and cold water (this is an ice plunge, and it will prevent the eggs from overcooking after they're removed from the hot water). Place a strainer in the sink next to the bowl of ice water.

When the timer goes off, pour the eggs into the strainer. Then, one by one, crack the eggshells gently against the sink and place in the cold water. Using your hands, move the eggs around in the ice water to stop them from cooking.

After about a minute, start peeling the eggs. I repeatedly dunk the eggs back in the ice water as I'm peeling them to help the shells come off. You can also hold them under the kitchen tap.

Sprinkle with salt and pepper and enjoy!

Egg Salad

Serves 4 to 6 • Batch Cook

As a busy surgeon, my dad didn't have a lot of time off. But when he did, he'd always take us to a place called Larry's Kosher Deli in New Jersey, which reminded him of his family's Russian-Jewish roots. We loved the deli's pastrami on rye, and we would get lots of egg salad and pickles. This is actually my mother's egg salad recipe, which my dad adored. Marjorie goes easy on the mayo, and a little heavier on the mustard, which is how I like it. Feel free to adjust it to your preferences.

6 Perfect Yellow Hard-Boiled Eggs (page 177), chopped (I use my hand chopper; makes it so easy)

2 tablespoons mayonnaise

2 teaspoons Dijon mustard

¼ teaspoon salt

⅛ teaspoon ground black pepper

½ teaspoon finely chopped fresh dill (optional)

1 teaspoon white wine vinegar

Place the eggs in a large bowl. Mix in the mayo, then the mustard. Add the salt, pepper, dill (if using), and vinegar and mix well. Taste and adjust the seasonings.

FYI

- When I batch cook this recipe, I use twelve eggs. It lasts in the fridge for a few days. I love making sandwiches with it, scooping it with vegetables, or using it as a dip with crackers.

Basic Chicken

Serves 4 (makes 8 cutlets) • Batch Cook

My mom made this all the time growing up; it was her standard recipe. I recently taught it on my YouTube channel, and a commenter said she'd made it for her son. The next night, when she tried a different dish, her kid asked, "Can you make that *Orange Is the New Black* lady's chicken again?" That made me laugh, and Marjorie would be very proud.

➤➤➤➤➤➤➤➤➤➤➤➤➤➤➤➤➤➤➤➤➤➤◀◀◀◀◀◀◀◀◀◀◀◀◀◀◀◀◀◀◀◀◀◀◀

4 chicken breasts

Salt and ground black pepper

Brown rice flour

1 tablespoon salted butter

1 tablespoon olive oil, plus more if needed

Chicken Broth (page 181)

➤➤➤➤➤➤➤➤➤➤➤➤➤➤➤➤➤➤➤➤➤➤◀◀◀◀◀◀◀◀◀◀◀◀◀◀◀◀◀◀◀◀◀◀◀

Place the chicken breasts between two sheets of parchment paper and pound them until they're about ¾ inch thick. Having the whole breast the same thickness allows it to cook more evenly. Pull off the top layer of parchment and discard it.

Season the chicken with salt and pepper. Evenly sprinkle with flour and pat it in lightly. Flip the chicken onto a fresh sheet of parchment and repeat on the other side.

In a large skillet, melt the butter in the oil over medium-high heat and add 1 tablespoon of broth. Add 2 chicken breasts (or whatever you can fit in your pan) and reduce the heat to medium. Cover and cook for 3 minutes, then take a peek. The outsides should start to turn white. Once the white really starts creeping up and over the edges, flip the cutlets. If the first bit of broth evaporates, add a little more.

Cover again and cook for 3 more minutes. The chicken should be done, but to make sure, cut one in half to take a look. Once it is white all the way through, it's done. Repeat with the remaining chicken, adding oil and butter as needed.

FYI

- This is a great protein grab to have in the fridge. Good for batch cooking, too! I use this in sandwiches and lettuce wraps or chopped in salads and soups. It's super versatile.

Chicken Broth

Makes about 3 quarts • Batch Cook, Freezer Friendly

You'll be amazed by how quick and easy it is to make broth. When I made a video of this recipe, we timed the preparation and it was *three minutes*. And a full minute of that was getting water from the tap!

>>>>>>>>>>>>>>>>>>>>>>><<<<<<<<<<<<<<<<<<<<<<<

1 (5-pound) organic chicken

2 medium carrots, scrubbed (peeled if you want) and cut into big chunks

A small handful of fresh thyme

A big sprig of fresh rosemary

1 medium yellow onion, coarsely chopped

2 large stalks celery, coarsely chopped

1 clove fermented black garlic, coarsely chopped (you can find it online or in better health food stores—it's my secret ingredient!)

2 bay leaves

2 teaspoons sea salt

2 teaspoons black peppercorns

>>>>>>>>>>>>>>>>>>>>>>><<<<<<<<<<<<<<<<<<<<<<<

Place all the ingredients in a large slow cooker (I use a 6.5 quart).* Fill with water almost to the top. Cook on high for the first four hours.

After 4 hours on high, the chicken meat should be cooked through. If you want to use the meat (I always do), carefully remove it from the submerged carcass using two forks. It should come off easily; if not, it's not cooked enough, in which case wait another hour. Be careful—the broth will be hot! Place the chicken meat in a glass container and store in the fridge to use in soups (like the one that follows), salads, sandwiches, and so on.

* I love using my slow cooker for this recipe, because I can just set it and step away. If you don't have one, you can definitely make broth in a pot on the stove, but it will need a little babysitting for safety.

Let the broth, with the carcass, continue to cook overnight or longer. Once I get the meat off the bones, I switch to low and cook for another 20 hours, for a total cook time of 24 hours.

Once the broth is finished cooking, let it cool until the slow cooker insert can be handled safely. Place a large fine-mesh strainer into a large soup pot and pour all the ingredients from the slow cooker into it. Shake the strainer to get as much of the broth out as possible. Discard the bones and other ingredients.

Let the broth cool completely, then refrigerate the whole pot or separate it into multiple glass containers. Once chilled, a soft layer of fat will form on the top of the broth. You can remove it carefully with a spoon or other tool, or leave it.

You can also freeze your broth in silicone ice cube trays for later use so you can pop them out to add flavor and nutrients to various dishes. Or you can freeze it in glass containers, but make sure the glass is tempered so it doesn't crack, and leave ½ inch of space at the top for expansion.

FAT SEPARATOR

If you'd like to use your broth immediately, you can remove the fat using a fat separator, a gadget my mother used frequently. The fat separator is coming back into style now that broths are big. Like a large a measuring cup, it has a long spout—coming out its side—that originates from the bottom inch of the cup (at least that's the design mine has; they vary). It works based on the premise that fat always rises to the top, so the spout pours broth, not fat. It's great!

Chicken Soup

Serves 6

I know chicken soup is famous for healing the sick, but we don't wait for a case of the sniffles to eat it in our household. I use the chicken pulled off the bones from my broth with some farmers market veggies, and it tastes amazing. I can feel it replenishing me almost immediately.

6 cups Chicken Broth (page 181) plus the leftover chicken meat, chopped

2 teaspoons chopped shallot

1 clove garlic, minced

1 teaspoons Bragg Liquid Aminos

½ teaspoon umeboshi plum vinegar

2 large carrots, peeled and sliced into ½-inch-thick half moons

2 stalks celery, strings removed,* sliced ½ inch thick

1 cup cooked brown rice

½ teaspoon chopped fresh dill

Salt and ground black pepper

Combine the broth, shallot, and garlic in a large pot. Add the liquid aminos and vinegar and bring to a boil over high heat. Reduce the heat and simmer for 3 to 5 minutes. Add the carrots and celery, cover, and cook for 5 to 10 minutes, until the vegetables are cooked through. Add the chicken, rice, and dill, season with salt and pepper, and serve.

* Celery string removal: Using your hands, "crack" one end of a stalk of celery (like you would a stick over your knee, but right at the end) and pull the broken bit down along the back of the stalk. All the strings will pull away from the stalk. Do the same thing from the other end, and the rest of the strings will pull away. You certainly don't have to do this, but I like to so the strings don't get stuck in my teeth.

Beef Broth

Makes about 3 quarts • Batch Cook, Freezer Friendly

I always assumed that making a great broth meant having to be a gourmet chef; that it was complicated or took years of experience to perfect. Turns out that's not the case! Beef broth is just as fast and easy as chicken broth. You should be able to put it together in a matter of minutes. Make sure the bones are organic and grass-fed.

>>>>>>>>>>>>>>>>>>>>><<<<<<<<<<<<<<<<<<<<<<<<

1 pound beef knuckle bones

1 pound beef short rib bones

1 pound beef marrow bones

2 large stalks celery, coarsely chopped

2 medium carrots, coarsely chopped

1 large onion, quartered

1 head garlic, unpeeled, sliced crosswise

1-inch piece ginger, sliced in half

1 clove fermented black garlic, cut in half

Small bunch fresh rosemary

Small bunch fresh thyme

2 bay leaves

2 teaspoons black peppercorns

2 teaspoons sea salt

>>>>>>>>>>>>>>>>>>>>><<<<<<<<<<<<<<<<<<<<<<<<

Give the bones a little rinse. Place all the ingredients in a large slow cooker (I use a 6.5 quart) and cover with water. Cook on low for 20 to 24 hours.

Let stand until the slow cooker insert is cool enough to handle. Place a large fine-mesh strainer into a large soup pot and strain the broth through it. Lift slightly and shimmy all the ingredients to get out all the golden goodness. Discard the bones and other ingredients.

Let the broth cool completely, then refrigerate the whole pot or separate it into multiple glass containers. Once chilled, a soft layer of fat will form on top of the broth. Run a knife all along the perimeter of the pot or storage container, lift the fat off of the broth, and discard it.

You can also freeze your broth in silicone ice cube trays for later use so you can pop them out to add flavor and nutrients to various dishes. Or you can freeze it in glass containers, but make sure the glass is tempered so it doesn't crack, and leave ½ inch of space at the top for expansion.

Turkey Burgers

Makes 8 big burgers • Batch Cook, Freezer Friendly, Trojan Food

These burgers are inspired by Dee, who would make much of her family's food—for the week—on Sunday and Monday, her days off. It's a great recipe for sneaking vegetables into kids!

I love to batch cook these burgers. I reheat them for sandwiches or chop them into salads or soups. They are super versatile.

>>>>>>>>>>>>>>>>>>>>>>>>><<<<<<<<<<<<<<<<<<<<<<<<<

1½ teaspoons salted butter, plus extra for cooking

1 tablespoon extra virgin olive oil, plus extra for cooking

¼ red bell pepper, seeded, peeled and finely chopped

1 clove garlic, finely chopped

1 shallot, finely chopped

½ medium zucchini, seeded and finely chopped

1 small carrot, finely chopped

¼ cup chopped fresh spinach

1 pound ground white turkey meat

1 pound ground dark turkey meat

2 teaspoons Worcestershire sauce

1 teaspoon salt

½ teaspoon ground black pepper

Chicken Broth (page 181)

>>>>>>>>>>>>>>>>>>>>>>>>><<<<<<<<<<<<<<<<<<<<<<<<<

In a large sauté pan, melt the butter in the oil over medium heat. Add the bell pepper, garlic, and shallot, turn the heat down to low, and cook until the shallot softens and becomes slightly translucent, about 5 minutes. Add the zucchini, carrot, and spinach and cook for 7 to 10 minutes, until all the vegetables are softened. Remove from the heat and let the vegetables cool.

In a large bowl, combine the turkey meat, Worcestershire sauce, salt, and black pepper. Add the cooked vegetables. Mix with your hands to combine the ingredients well, but beware of overmixing, which will make the burgers mushy.

Remove a large meatball-size handful and gently mold it into a ball, then press down on it in the palm of your hand to flatten it into a ¾-inch-high patty. Continue molding it around the edges, if you like. Finish with the rest of the meat mixture.

In a large skillet, heat 1½ teaspoons butter and about 1½ teaspoons oil over medium heat. Place four of the burgers in the hot oil, making sure they don't touch one another. Drop 1 tablespoon chicken broth into the pan, in the middle space between the burgers. Cover, reduce the heat to medium-low, and let cook/steam for 3 minutes. You'll have to keep an eye on the temperature; if it starts to sizzle too loudly, turn down the heat.

Flip the burgers. Add another tablespoon of broth, if needed. Cook for 3 more minutes. If you're not sure whether they're cooked through, press one with your finger; if the burger is firm, it should be done. Slice one open to double check. Remove the first batch of burgers and set aside.

Lower the heat to low, as the pan will be very hot from the first batch of burgers. Add more butter and oil as needed. Place the remaining burgers in the pan and add 1 tablespoon broth. Turn the heat up to medium-low and cook the second batch of burgers following the instructions above.

Serve hot, on buns, in lettuce cups, or just plain. If you're keeping some for later, let them cool and store in a glass container in the fridge.

Oven-Roasted Frozen Salmon with Asparagus and Baby Potatoes

Serves 4

Inspired by Amber, I like this recipe because I get so upset when I buy wild-caught fish, don't end up using it, and it goes bad. But with this recipe, I can just put it in the freezer and not worry about that. I love any recipe that can take frozen food and make it taste great! Amber loves it for two reasons: "First, I don't always have time to buy fresh fish, so having a whole bag of frozen fish, ready to go, is incredibly helpful. Second, this recipe is easy and—most important—quick!"

>>>>>>>>>>>>>>>>>>>>><<<<<<<<<<<<<<<<<<<<<<

4 frozen wild-caught salmon fillets	Salt
1 shallot	Ground black pepper
2 cloves garlic	4 tablespoons olive oil
1 tablespoon Champagne vinegar	1½ pounds baby potatoes, cut in half
½ teaspoon paprika	
Juice of ½ lemon	1 bunch asparagus
1 teaspoon maple syrup	Chopped Italian flat-leaf parsley for garnish
½ teaspoon Dijon mustard	

>>>>>>>>>>>>>>>>>>>>><<<<<<<<<<<<<<<<<<<<<<

Preheat the oven to 350°F.

In a blender, combine the shallot, garlic, vinegar, paprika, lemon juice, maple syrup, mustard, ¼ teaspoon salt, a few grinds of black pepper, and 2 tablespoons of the oil and blend. It should be on the thicker side and slightly chunky so the sauce does not completely run off the fish.

Remove the fish from the freezer, but do not thaw it. Place the fish in a casserole dish and cover the dish with tinfoil.

Meanwhile, toss the baby potatoes in 1 tablespoon of the remaining oil, a sprinkle of salt, and a few grinds of pepper. Break off the hard ends of the asparagus and toss them in the remaining 1 tablespoon oil. Season like potatoes with salt and pepper. Lay the potatoes on half of a large baking sheet.

Put the salmon and potatoes in the oven and bake for 15 minutes. Pull back the tinfoil from the casserole dish, pour the sauce over the salmon, and make a few stabs with a knife into the fish so the sauce can be absorbed. Re-close the tinfoil. Stir the potatoes and add the asparagus to the other side of the baking sheet.

After another 15 to 20 minutes, check everything for doneness: It's ready when a fork easily goes through the potatoes, the asparagus is tender but still crisp, and the fish is opaque in the middle.

Plate the salmon with the potatoes and asparagus. Salt and pepper to taste. Sprinkle parsley over salmon. Enjoy!

VARIATIONS

- Amber batches this recipe and uses it for a cold salmon salad the next day.
- Sometimes I will slice and reheat the fish on low with my lunch; you can also add it to a sandwich.

KIDS' FOOD

Turkey Meatball Soup

Serves 4 • Trojan Food

This recipe is inspired by Mila, who shares: "I have a great mom. She wants to be super involved and she also happens to be an unbelievable cook. So, my husband and I devised a plan where we make her cook for our children and she loves it! That's a really good family hack. Make your in-laws cook!" Mila is also a huge fan of bone broth for its high nutrition content, and her mom makes their family a lot of soups. This is a turkey meatball soup that's easy to make and so cozy and yummy.

SOUP

8 cups Chicken Broth (page 181)

2 tablespoons Bragg Liquid Aminos

2 tablespoons umeboshi plum vinegar

1 large carrot, thinly sliced

1 large stalk celery, strings removed (see page 183), thinly sliced

1-inch piece ginger, cut in half

1 cup dried brown rice rotini noodles (2 ounces)

2 stalks bok choy, cut into 1-inch chunks

MEATBALLS

1 tablespoon salted butter

½ teaspoon toasted sesame oil

¼ medium yellow onion, minced

1 clove garlic, minced

8 ounces ground white turkey meat

½ cup breadcrumbs, store-bought or homemade

1 large egg, beaten

1½ teaspoons Bragg Liquid Aminos

1 teaspoon hoisin sauce

TO MAKE THE SOUP

In a large saucepan, combine the broth, liquid aminos, vinegar, carrot, celery, and ginger and bring to a boil over high heat. Cover and reduce the heat to maintain a simmer.

In a separate saucepan, cook the noodles according to the instructions on the package. Pour the noodles through a strainer, then move them to a bowl of fresh water and set aside (this prevents the noodles from sticking together).

TO MAKE THE MEATBALLS

Meanwhile, in a small skillet, melt the butter in the oil over medium-low heat. Add the onion and garlic and stir until translucent, about 5 minutes. Transfer to a large bowl. Add the turkey, breadcrumbs, egg, liquid aminos, and hoisin sauce. Mix with your hands until just combined and shape into 1-inch balls.

Add the meatballs to the simmering broth, raise the heat, and bring back to a boil. Reduce the heat, cover, and simmer for about 15 minutes, until the meat is no longer pink, adding the bok choy 5 minutes before the timer goes off. Strain the noodles and add them to the broth. Remove and discard the ginger.

FYI

- I like to add pickled Persian cucumbers as a crunchy side (see page 200). Instead of dill, add some red pepper flakes and a dash of toasted sesame oil.

Chicken Tenders

Serves 4 to 6 • Batch Cook, Freezer Friendly

Daphne shared this recipe as a go-to with her family, and I make it all the time. Chicken tenders are obviously great for eating immediately, but they can be batched, frozen (if they last that long!), and reheated. You can also make them with a flaky white fish like cod—just reduce the cooking time a little.

> ≫≫≫≫≫≫≫≫≫≫≫≫≫≫≫≫≪≪≪≪≪≪≪≪≪≪≪≪≪≪≪≪≪

4 chicken breasts

2 cups brown rice flour

1 to 2 teaspoons garlic salt

3 large eggs

2 teaspoons soy sauce

2 cups breadcrumbs
(preferably homemade)

1 teaspoon dried oregano

1 teaspoon all-purpose
chicken seasoning

¾ cup olive oil, plus extra if needed

> ≫≫≫≫≫≫≫≫≫≫≫≫≫≫≫≫≪≪≪≪≪≪≪≪≪≪≪≪≪≪≪≪≪

Lay the chicken breasts in between two layers of parchment paper. Pound evenly until each breast is about ¾ inch thick. Cut into desired shapes, such as strips or circles.

Set out three large bowls. Mix the flour with garlic salt in one bowl. Beat the eggs with the soy sauce in the second bowl. Mix the breadcrumbs with the oregano and all-purpose chicken seasoning in the third bowl.

Place a chicken cutlet in the flour mixture, then into the egg wash, then into the breadcrumbs. Gently pat the breadcrumbs onto both sides. Continue with the rest of the chicken.

Heat the oil in a large skillet over medium-high heat. (This is a shallow fry: more oil than if you were sautéing, but less than covering a whole piece of chicken. You want the oil frying about three quarters of the way up the sides of the chicken cutlet.) If you are using a smaller pan, use less oil. Carefully place as much chicken in the pan as fits without overcrowding; it should start sizzling and bubbling right away. Reduce the heat to medium-low, being sure to maintain a nice sizzling bubble around the cutlets.

Cover and cook for 3 minutes, or until the chicken is starting to turn white and the breadcrumbs brown around the edges. Flip and cook for another 3 minutes, or until the chicken is white all the way through.

Transfer to a cooling rack with paper towels beneath it to catch any oil drippings. Continue cooking the rest of the chicken in batches and serve.

VARIATIONS

- Daphne likes to add pecorino cheese in with the breadcrumbs to change up the recipe. She also has a different version in her book *The Happy Cook* that uses almonds instead of breadcrumbs to make it Paleo, but she says they don't hold up as well for freezing and reheating.
- This recipe can be baked instead of fried. Place on a parchment-lined baking sheet and bake in a preheated 350°F degree oven for 20 to 25 minutes.

FYI

- For freezing, layer the cutlets in between sheets of parchment paper, put into a storage container, and freeze. To reheat, place in a preheated 350°F oven until heated through.
- I like to make breadcrumbs from the bread in the Mezze Platter (page 201) that's a couple of days old. They stick amazingly to the chicken and turn so golden and crunchy as they cook!

IT'S ALL ABOUT BRANDING, BABY!

When it comes to feeding kids, Jenji says that marketing is everything, and many of the Mom Squad agree. To a five-year-old an egg can be pretty boring, but what if it's a pizza egg? Or a spinach . . . cupcake? If your kid's a picky eater, don't be afraid to get all Disney on her and whip out the Princess Pasta and Tigger Toast. P.S.: This only works until about age seven. After that, we'll need some luck!

Oven-Roasted Chicken and Veggie "Stir Fry"

Serves 4 to 6

I made this recipe by accident, and it has become a staple in our house. It's so easy, and one of the things I love about it is that I can prep it in the morning, and when I get home from work, I pop it in the oven. An hour and a half later, we have dinner!

1 medium head cauliflower, cut into florets

1 medium head broccoli, cut into florets

1 medium white onion, sliced

4 medium carrots, sliced into ½-inch rounds

6 cloves garlic, thinly sliced

2 tablespoons Bragg Liquid Aminos, plus extra if needed

2 teaspoons umeboshi plum vinegar

2 tablespoons toasted sesame oil, plus extra if needed

1 (3½-pound) whole chicken

2 tablespoons salted butter

Salt and ground black pepper

½ lemon, quartered

Brown rice or brown rice noodles for serving

Preheat the oven to 350°F.

In a roasting pan, combine the cauliflower, broccoli, onion, carrots, and 2 cloves of the sliced garlic. Add the liquid aminos, vinegar, and sesame oil and toss well.

Rinse and pat the chicken dry. Slide your fingers between the skin and the meat to separate slightly. Slide ½ tablespoon of butter, plus 1 clove of the remaining sliced garlic between the skin and the meat on each side. Season the cavity of the chicken with salt and pepper, then add the lemon and the remaining two cloves of garlic. Tie the legs together and wrap cooking twine around the chicken, holding the legs close to the body. Rub the entire chicken with the remaining tablespoon of the butter, then rub in 1 teaspoon salt and ½ teaspoon pepper.

Place the chicken directly on top of the vegetables in the center. Lay a piece of parchment paper on top of the chicken and cover the entire pan with tinfoil, cinching the sides tightly all around. Bake for 1 hour, then remove the tinfoil and parchment paper and bake for another 30 minutes, or until the chicken is cooked through or measures 165° on a meat thermometer inserted into the thigh.

Remove the roasting pan from the oven. Once the chicken has cooled a bit, pull all of the meat from the bones. I usually discard the skin. Place the pieces of meat into the roasting pan and mix with the roasted vegetables. Place the roasting pan on the stovetop over medium-low heat and stir all the ingredients together like a stir-fry. Add a few dashes of sesame oil and liquid aminos, if needed.

Serve hot over brown rice or brown rice noodles.

VARIATION
Try this with autumn veggies like winter squash and root vegetables. It's sweet, cozy, and satisfying.

Creamy Pasta Primavera with Chicken Sausage

Serves 4 or more • Trojan Food

Jill makes a version of this recipe for her family when she's got lots of vegetables and little time. It's fast, nutritious, and delicious. And she's careful not to get rigid about this recipe: "We joke that it never tastes the same twice because we never have the same vegetables! Whatever you have hanging around in your veggie drawer . . . celery, bits of fennel, it doesn't matter at all. Just start with the longest-cooking vegetables and move to the quickest."

➤➤➤➤➤➤➤➤➤➤➤➤➤➤➤➤➤➤➤➤➤➤➤➤➤➤➤➤➤➤➤➤➤➤➤➤➤➤➤

2 to 4 organic chicken sausages

2 tablespoons olive oil

2 cloves garlic, minced

½ medium yellow onion, cut into medium dice

1 large carrot, cut in thin diagonal slices

1 small zucchini, cut in thin diagonal slices

1 cup small broccoli florets

½ cup cut green beans in 1-inch lengths

Salt and ground black pepper

8 ounces uncooked brown rice pasta (I like spirals by the Bionaturae brand)

1 teaspoon salted butter

2 to 4 ounces goat cheese, crumbled

Parmesan cheese (optional)

➤➤➤➤➤➤➤➤➤➤➤➤➤➤➤➤➤➤➤➤➤➤➤➤➤➤➤➤➤➤➤➤➤➤➤➤➤➤➤

Cook the sausages in a large skillet over medium heat according to the directions on the package until crispy and cooked through, typically 10 to 15 minutes. Remove from the pan to a plate and set aside.

As the sausage is cooking, chop the vegetables and bring a large pot of water to a rolling boil.

Allow the pan used for the sausages to cool a little. Turn the heat to medium-low and add the oil, garlic, and onion. Cook for about 5 minutes, enough to soften the onion. Add the carrot, stirring regularly to avoid burning. When the carrot seems softened, after about 3 minutes, add the zucchini, broccoli, and green beans. Season generously with salt and pepper and stir well so the newer vegetables get a little oil on them and soften slightly, about 5 minutes. Dribble ¼ cup water into the skillet, raise the heat to medium-high (this will create steam), cover, and let the vegetables cook for 3 more minutes.

Cook the pasta according to the directions on the box and drain. Transfer to a bowl, add the butter, and stir.

Chop the sausages into bite-size pieces. Remove the vegetables from the heat and place them in a large bowl. Add the sausages, pasta, and crumbled goat cheese. Toss gently so the goat cheese melts a bit and coats the noodles. Finish with some salt and pepper and Parmesan cheese, if desired. Serve hot.

ROMANTIC DINNER OPTIONS

Stovetop Cod with Baby Potatoes, Quick Pickles, and Cherry Tomato Relish

Serves 2

This meal is based on one that my husband and I enjoyed on a trip a couple of years ago. It is a fantastic combination of flavors and textures, and yet so simple! I used to find cooking fish sort of daunting, because I didn't want it to smell up my entire home. I like fish recipes that trap the smell and have easy cleanup, and this one does just that! If you choose to make all the dishes as a meal, begin with the potatoes, followed by pickles, relish, and fish.

Stovetop Cod

>>>>>>>>>>>>>>>>>>>>><<<<<<<<<<<<<<<<<<<<<<<<

2 (8-ounce) boneless cod fillets

Juice of ½ lemon, plus wedges for serving

Olive oil

1 teaspoon salt

½ teaspoon ground black pepper

½ teaspoon chopped Italian flat-leaf parsley (optional)

1 tablespoon of butter

>>>>>>>>>>>>>>>>>>>>><<<<<<<<<<<<<<<<<<<<<<<<

Rinse the fish and pat it dry. Place the fish onto a piece of parchment-lined tinfoil.* Squeeze lemon juice onto the fillets, spreading it with your fingers. Drizzle with oil and massage it into the fillets. Sprinkle with the salt and pepper.

---

* This is just a personal preference of mine; the jury is still out on whether tinfoil leaches aluminum into food at high heats. To be safe, I place the fish on a smaller piece of parchment inside the tinfoil.

Lift two opposite sides of the tinfoil and bring them together, first folding them together and then rolling them down, like a paper lunch bag, leaving a couple of inches of room above the fish. Fold up the two sides, then fold down and pinch the tinfoil so it's sealed and no juices can leak out. The tinfoil will look like a little pouch with air above the fish, so the fish can steam within it.

Place the pouches in a large sauté pan over medium-high heat. As soon as you hear some sizzle from within the pouches, reduce the heat to medium-low. Gently cover with a lid. Unless you have a domed lid, it will rest on top of the pouches and may not make contact with the sides of the sauté pan, which is fine. As the sizzle gets louder, reduce the heat even lower. Cook for 6 to 8 minutes, until the fish is flaky and cooked through.

Remove the pouches from the pan and open them carefully. With a spatula, lift the fish from the pouches and transfer to a plate. Discard the parchment and tinfoil. Place ½ tablespoon butter onto each fish filet and let it melt. Garnish with parsley (if using) and lemon wedges and serve.

VARIATIONS
- Use any fish you like; simply adjust the cooking time according to thickness.
- Try other toppings like olives, capers, and other herbs.

Baby Potatoes

>>>>>>>>>>>>>>>>>>>>>>>><<<<<<<<<<<<<<<<<<<<<<<<<

12 baby potatoes	Butter
Salt and ground black pepper	

>>>>>>>>>>>>>>>>>>>>>>>><<<<<<<<<<<<<<<<<<<<<<<<<

Rinse the potatoes well. Steam or boil them until tender and easily punctured with a fork, about 20 minutes. Drain. Add salt, pepper, and butter to taste.

Quick Pickles

4 Persian cucumbers, cut diagonally into ¾-inch slices

½ teaspoon chopped fresh dill

1 to 2 tablespoons umeboshi plum vinegar

Mix the cucumbers and dill in a small bowl or jar and drizzle with vinegar. Massage until well coated. Let sit for 20 minutes, then drain excess vinegar. These pickles will keep refrigerated for about 3 days.

Cherry Tomato Relish

1 teaspoon salted butter

1 tablespoon olive oil

1 clove garlic, finely chopped

1 tablespoon finely chopped red onion

1 teaspoon turbinado sugar

1 teaspoon white wine vinegar

Generous pinch of sea salt

Generous pinch of ground black pepper

10 to 12 cherry tomatoes, coarsely chopped

Place the butter and oil in an unheated medium skillet and add the garlic and onion. Place over medium heat and stir. Once it starts sizzling, reduce the heat to low and cook until the onions are translucent, 5 to 7 minutes.

Add the sugar, vinegar, salt, and pepper and cook, stirring, until the sugar dissolves. Add the cherry tomatoes, increase the heat to medium-low, cover, and cook for 3 to 5 minutes. I like my relish to have a bit of texture, so I cook the tomatoes for the shorter amount of time. It you want them softer, cook for the full 5 minutes. Remove from the heat and let cool to room temperature. Serve as a relish with the fish.

Mezze Platter

Bread recipe makes 2 large loaves

This meal is my easy spin on a mezze platter. A great loaf of bread with a bunch of little noshies, and cheese arranged on a cutting board . . . yum! I throw this together when I have a loaf of my Go-to Gluten-Free Bread prepared (my favorite gluten-free bread recipe ever!).

There used to be a bakery near me called Jennifer's Way that used only organic and gluten-free ingredients. It made a bread that I loved. The bakery ultimately shut down, much to my dismay, but I found the recipe in a cookbook of the same title. I've tweaked it a bit, but this recipe is very much inspired by that original bread I used to long for.

If you pair this platter with some good wine, it makes a great date-night dinner!

>>>>>>>>>>>>>>>>>>>>>>><<<<<<<<<<<<<<<<<<<<<<<<<<

FOR THE BREAD:

2 cups warm filtered water

⅓ cup olive oil

2 tablespoons raw honey

1 tablespoon maple syrup

2 teaspoons apple cider vinegar

2 tablespoons active dry yeast

¼ cup chia seeds

1½ cups room-temperature water

2 cups millet flour

1½ cups sorghum flour

½ cup brown rice flour

1 cup cornstarch

½ cup arrowroot powder

1½ cups potato starch

1½ tablespoons xanthan gum

2 teaspoons sea salt

½ cup all-purpose gluten-free flour

FOR THE PLATTER:

Toasted and buttered slices of Go-to Gluten-Free Bread (if the bread is fresh, you don't have to toast it)

Hummus

Carrot sticks

Celery sticks

Mini sweet peppers

Sliced Persian cucumbers

Kalamata olives

Cheese (your favorite)

Nuts (almonds, walnuts, Brazil nuts, or any of your favorites)

Sliced meats of your choice

>>>>>>>>>>>>>>>>>>>>><<<<<<<<<<<<<<<<<<<<<<<<

GO-TO GLUTEN-FREE BREAD

Preheat the oven to 375°F. Line a baking sheet with parchment paper.

In a small bowl, mix the warm water, oil, honey, maple syrup, and vinegar. Add the yeast and set aside for 10 minutes. (It should become foamy after a minute, which means the yeast is activating.)

In a separate bowl, mix the chia seeds with the room-temperature water and set aside.

In a stand mixer fitted with the paddle attachment, mix the millet flour, sorghum flour, brown rice flour, cornstarch, arrowroot, potato starch, xanthan gum, and salt until just combined. Add the yeast mixture and chia seed mixture. Mix for 2 to 3 minutes, until fully combined. Mix in the all-purpose gluten-free flour, until fully integrated.

With your hands, shape the dough into two equal sections on the baking sheet (the dough will stick to your hands). Wet your hands to shape into two oval loaves. Score the top of the bread with a knife.

Bake for 40 to 50 minutes, until the temperature reaches 200°F. I use a meat thermometer to check. Let the bread cool completely before cutting into it (it continues to cook after you take it out of the oven before cooling).

VARIATION

This bread is a great base to add fillings to. When Angela was about to become a mother, she shared with me a profound moment for her: "My mom had given me a cookbook, and I was like, 'I am going to cook something for my family!' I made olive bread. It was the first time I sensed this weird primal feeling . . . this primal mothering instinct." Inspired by Angela, I tried a version of this bread with chopped olives and rosemary! It is delicious and a great addition to the mezze platter.

THE PLATTER

Build your platter on top of a big wooden cutting board: Lay out the sliced bread along one side, then make little piles of all the other ingredients around the board. If you don't have a big board, you can use a serving platter.

Aperol Spritz

Makes 1 drink

When Ben and I took our first vacation in more than two years, we chose a warm island destination. I'm not usually a sun seeker, considering I've been nicknamed Elvira in the past, but this particular trip was amazing. One of the cocktails we had there was an Aperol spritz. I'd had Aperol before, but something about this particular combination, plus being on a vacation, made it even yummier. Every time I have this cocktail now, I am reminded of that special trip with my husband.

>>>>>>>>>>>>>>>>>>>>><<<<<<<<<<<<<<<<<<<<<<

1 part Aperol   1 part club soda

1 part Brut Champagne

>>>>>>>>>>>>>>>>>>>>><<<<<<<<<<<<<<<<<<<<<<

Combine all the ingredients in wine glass filled with ice. Enjoy!

Strawberries Dipped in Chocolate

Makes about 12

This is a special treat for a romantic night. Fast and easy but memorable and sexy.

>>>>>>>>>>>>>>>>>>>>>><<<<<<<<<<<<<<<<<<<<<<<<

1 pint strawberries

1 cup semisweet chocolate chips

1 tablespoon coconut oil

>>>>>>>>>>>>>>>>>>>>>><<<<<<<<<<<<<<<<<<<<<<<<

Line a baking sheet with parchment paper.

Rinse the strawberries, pat them dry, and set aside. Do not remove the tops.

Melt the chocolate chips with the oil in a heatproof glass bowl nestled into a pot containing about 1 inch of boiling water (or in a double boiler). Make sure the bowl doesn't touch the water. Stir until the chocolate and oil are melted and integrated. Turn off the heat.

Dip the strawberries into the chocolate, letting any excess drip off, and place on the prepared baking sheet. Refrigerate for about 30 minutes to allow the chocolate to set.

Let the strawberries sit at room temperature for a few minutes before serving.

VARIATIONS
- Garnish the dipped strawberries with Maldon sea salt.
- Swap in white chocolate chips and garnish with colored sprinkles.

A Final Word...

As we continue this journey of discovery together, may our hearts expand and our wisdom deepen. When we find ourselves around kitchen tables, at our sit spots, blinking through sleepless nights, let's remember: We are in this thing together.

Wishing us all health, happiness, and the greatest nutrition of all . . . love.

A mother is a lighthouse
And there are rocks everywhere.
She will guide you the best way she knows how.
A mother is there when you need light
And will throw it in your direction.
But the weather shifts and the winds will change;
There will be sunny days and impossible storms
And life will happen to you
And your little boat.
The mother stands as tall as she can
Through the fog.

LAURA

NOTES

INTRODUCTION: A NEW KIND OF "PLUS ONE"
1. Lucy Lamble, "With 250 Babies Born Each Minute, How Many People Can the Earth Sustain?," *The Guardian*, April 23, 2018, https://www.theguardian.com/global-development/2018/apr/23population-how-many-people-can-the-earth-sustain-lucy-lamble.

CHAPTER 3: YOU, VERSION 2.0, MOM EDITION
1. University of Denver Department of Psychology, https://www.du.edu/ahss/psychology/facultystaffstudents/faculty-listing/kim.html.

2. Jorge Barazza et al., "Oxytocin Infusion Increases Charitable Donations Regardless of Monetary Resources," *Hormones and Behavior* 60, no. 2 (May 2011): 148–51, https://www.researchgate.net/publication/51149904_Oxytocin_infusion_increases_charitable_donations_regardless_of_monetary_resources.

3. Rita Watson, MPH, "Oxytocin: The Love and Trust Hormone Can Be Deceptive," *Psychology Today*, October 14, 2013, https://www.psychologytoday.com/us/blog/love-and-gratitude/201310/oxytocin-the-love-and-trust-hormone-can-be-deceptive.

4. Louann Brizendine, *The Female Brain* (New York: Broadway Books, 2006), 101–103.

CHAPTER 4: CONTROL
1. Richard Adams, "Having a Working Mother Works for Daughters," *The Guardian*, June 24, 2015, https://www.theguardian.com/world/2015/jun/24/having-a-working-mother-works-for-daughters.

CHAPTER 5: STRESS
1. Norman B. Schmidt et al., "Exploring Human Freeze Responses to a Threat Stressor," *Journal of Behavior Therapy and Experimental Psychiatry* 39, no. 3 (September 2008): 292–304, https://www.ncbi.nlm.nih.gov/pmc/articles/PMC2489204/.

2. Shelley E. Taylor et al., "Behavioral Responses to Stress in Females: Tend and Befriend, Not Fight-or-Flight," *Psychological Review* 107, no. 3 (2000): 411–29, https://taylorlab.psych.ucla.edu/wp-content/uploads/sites/5/2014/10/2000_Biobehavioral-responses-to-stress-in-females_tend-and-befriend.pdf.

3. "It's Official: Spending Time Outside Is Good for You," *Science Daily*, July 6, 2018, https://www.sciencedaily.com/releases/2018/07/180706102842.htm.

4. Sandee LaMotte, "Hillary Clinton Uses Alternate Nostril Breathing. Should You?," CNN Health, September 14, 2017, https://www.cnn.com/2017/09/14/health/hillary-clinton-alternate-nostril-breathing/index.html.

5. Waleed O. Twal, Amy E. Wahlquist, and Sundaravadivel Balasubramanian, "Yogic Breathing When Compared to Attention Control Reduces the Levels of Pro-inflammatory Biomarkers in Saliva: A Pilot Randomized Controlled Trial," *BMC Complementary and Alternative Medicine* 16 (August 2016), https://bmccomplementalternmed.biomedcentral.com/articles/10.1186/s12906-016-1286-87.

6. "Yoga for Anxiety and Depression," Harvard Health Publishing, Harvard Medical School, updated May 9, 2018, https://www.health.harvard.edu/mind-and-mood/yoga-for-anxiety-and-depression.

7. "Why Do We Sleep, Anyway?," Harvard Medical School, Division of Sleep Medicine, last reviewed December 2007, https://www.health.harvard.edu/mind-and-mood/yoga-for-anxiety-and-depression.

8. Mayo Clinic Staff, "Exercise and Stress: Get Moving to Manage Stress," Mayo Clinic, March 8, 2018, https://www.mayoclinic.org/healthy-lifestyle/stress-management/in-depth/exercise-and-stress/art-20044469.

9. Amy Yang, Abraham A. Palmer, and Harriet de Wit, "Genetics of Caffeine Consumption and Responses to Coffee," *Psychopharmacology* 211, no. 3 (August 2010): 245–57, https://www.ncbi.nlm.nih.gov/pmc/articles/PMC4242593/.

CHAPTER 6: MOTHERHOOD AROUND THE WORLD

1. Pamela Druckerman, *Bringing Up Bébé: One American Mother Discovers the Wisdom of French Parenting* (New York: Penguin, 2012), 278.

2. Michaeleen Doucleff, "Secrets of a Maya Supermom: What Parenting Books Don't Tell You," WBGO.org, May 11, 2018, https://www.wbgo.org/post/best-mothers-day-gift-get-mom-out-box#stream/0.

CHAPTER 7: COMMUNITY

1. Louann Brizendine, *The Female Brain* (New York: Broadway Books, 2006), 36–37.

2. Melissa G. Hunt, "No More FOMO: Limiting Social Media Decreases Loneliness and Depression," *Journal of Social and Clinical Psychology* 37, no 10 (2018): 751–68.

3. Leslie J. Seltzer, "Instant Messages vs. Speech: Hormones and Why We Still Need to Hear Each Other," *Evolution and Human Behavior* 33, no. 1 (January 2012): 42–45, https://www.ncbi.nlm.nih.gov/pmc/articles/PMC3277914/.

4. William M. Kenkel, Allison M. Perkeybile, and C. Sue Carter, "The Neurobiological Causes and Effects of Alloparenting," *Developmental Neurobiology* 77, no. 2 (February 2017): 214–32, https://www.ncbi.nlm.nih.gov/pmc/articles/PMC5768312/.

CHAPTER 8: KEEPING THE LOVE ALIVE

1. Jamie Ducharme, "'Phubbing' Is Hurting Your Relationships. Here's What It Is," *Time*, March 28, 2018, https://time.com/5216853/what-is-phubbing/.

CHAPTER 10: LET'S TALK FOOD

1. Charles M. Benbrook, "Trends in Glyphosate Herbicide Use in the United States and Globally," *Environmental Sciences Europe* 28, no. 1 (2016): 3, https://www.ncbi.nlm.nih.gov/pmc/articles/PMC5044953/.

2. "Estimated Annual Agricultural Pesticide Use," U.S. Geological Survey, Dept. of the Interior, Pesticide National Synthesis Project, 2016, https://water.usgs.gov/nawqa/pnsp/usage/maps/show_map.php?year=2016&map=GLYPHOSATE&hilo=L&disp= Glyphosate.

3. "Recent Trends in GE Adoption," U.S. Dept. of Agriculture, Economic Research Service, updated September 18, 2019, https://www.ers.usda.gov/data-products/adoption-of-genetically-engineered-crops-in-the-us/recent-trends-in-ge-adoption.aspx.

4. "Sugars and Sweeteners: Background," U.S. Dept. of Agriculture, Economic Research Service, updated August 20, 2019, https://www.ers.usda.gov/topics/crops/sugar-sweeteners/background.aspx.

5. Global Glyphosate Study, https://glyphosatestudy.org/.

6. Vanessa Romo, "Roundup Weed Killer Could Be Linked to Widespread Bee Deaths," NPR Science, September 25, 2018, https://www.npr.org/2018/09/25/651618685/study-roundup-weed-killer-could-be-linked-to-widespread-bee-deaths.

7. Awad A. Shehata et al., "The Effect of Glyphosate on Potential Pathogens and Beneficial Members of Poultry Microbiota in Vitro," *Current Microbiology* 66, no. 4 (April 2013): 350–58, https://www.ncbi.nlm.nih.gov/pubmed/23224412.

8. Anthony Samsell and Stephanie Seneff, "Glyphosate, Pathways to Modern Diseases II: Celiac Sprue and Gluten Intolerance," *Interdisciplinary Toxicology* 6, no. 4 (December 2013): 159–84, https://www.ncbi.nlm.nih.gov/pmc/articles/PMC3945755/.

9. Qixing Mao et al., "The Ramazzini Institute 13-Week Pilot Study on Glyphosate and Roundup Administered at Human-Equivalent Dose to Sprague Dawley Rats: Effects on the Microbiome," *Environmental Health* 17 (2018): 50, https://www.ncbi.nlm.nih.gov/pmc/articles/PMC5972442/.

10. "Inflammatory Bowel Disease Diagnoses Rising," *Discovery's Edge: Mayo Clinic's Research Magazine*, February 20, 2017, https://discoverysedge.mayo.edu/2017/02/20/inflammatory-bowel-disease-diagnoses-rising/; Tara Parker Pope, "Celiac Disease Becoming More Common," *Well* (blog), *New York Times*, July 2, 2009, https://well.blogs.nytimes.com/2009/07/02/celiac-disease-becoming-more-common/; "Food Allergy 101: Facts and Statistics," Food Allergy Research & Education, n.d., https://www.foodallergy.org/life-with-food-allergies/food-allergy-101/facts-and-statistics; Guifeng Xu et al., "Twenty-Year Trends in Diagnosed Attention-Deficit/Hyperactivity Disorder Among US Children and Adolescents, 1997–2016," *JAMA Network Open* 1, no. 4 (August 2018), https://jamanetwork.com/journals/jamanetworkopen/fullarticle/2698633; Stacy Simon, "Obesity Rates Continue to Rise Among Adults in the US," American Cancer Society, April 6, 2018, https://www.cancer.org/latest-news/obesity-rates-continue-to-rise-among-adults-in-the-us.html; and Grace Rattue, "Autoimmune Disease Rates Increasing," *Medical News Today*, June 22, 2012, https://www.medicalnewstoday.com/articles/246960.php.

11. Richard Gonzales, "California Jury Awards $2 Billion to Couple in Roundup Weed Killer Cancer Trial," NPR Business, May 13, 2019, https://www.npr.org/2019/05/13/723056453/california-jury-awards-2-billion-to-couple-in-roundup-weed-killer-cancer-trial.

12. Emily Laurence, "Watch Out, Whole Foods: How Costco Became the Most Important Player in the Organic Produce Game," *Well + Good*, February 27, 2017, https://www.wellandgood.com/good-food/costco-certified-organic-produce-expansion/slide/3/.

13. Christine Michel Carter, "Millennial Moms: The $2.4 Trillion Social Media Influencer," *Forbes*, June 15, 2017, https://www.forbes.com/sites/christinecarter/2017/06/15/millennial-moms-the-2-4-trillion-social-media-influencer/#429198d02261.

14. Julia Moskin, "Bones, Broth, Bliss," *New York Times*, January 7, 2015, https://www.nytimes.com/2015/01/07/dining/bone-broth-evolves-from-prehistoric-food-to-paleo-drink.html.

ACKNOWLEDGMENTS

Ben: My Husband, my Love, my Lighthouse. Thank you for your support, creativity, and love. Thank you for your *You.* You are a force and inspire me every day. I love you beyond . . .

Ella: You opened my eyes to a world and a love I didn't know was possible. Being your mother is the truest gift. You are my heart.

The Mom Squad: Thank you for sharing your wisdom and insight. We will all benefit from your beautiful contributions.

Rebecca Kaplan, Diane Shaw, and my team at Abrams: Thank you for believing in me and this book. I so appreciate your hard work and collaboration in bringing this book to life. I can't wait for what's to come.

Gillian and Steven Foster: Your support and care means so much to me. I am grateful for your wisdom and guidance.

Mommy and the Prepon Family: Thank you for always supporting me. Mommy, thank you for walking to the beat of your own drum and inspiring us to do the same.

Jessica Porter: Thank you for your guidance, collaboration, and contributions to this book. I am so grateful for your wisdom, kindness, and humor. Thank you for helping me bring this book to fruition.

Folio Literary Management: Frank and Dado, thank you for believing in my vision and for helping me get my book to Rebecca and the Abrams team. I look forward to what's to come and thank you for being with me on this journey.

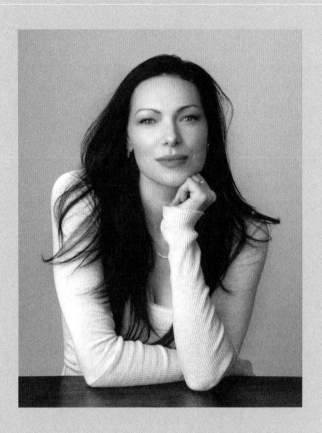

Laura Prepon is a versatile actress whose career spans both film and television. She made her television debut on the long-running sitcom *That '70s Show*, portraying Donna Pinciotti, and recently wrapped the seventh season of the hit Netflix original series *Orange Is the New Black*, on which she portrayed Alex Vause. In addition to her on-camera work in *Orange Is the New Black*, Laura directed multiple episodes. She is also the *New York Times* bestselling author of *The Stash Plan*.